INVISIBLE PAIN,
UNSTOPPABLE POWER

Foreword by Dr. John Demartini
Human Behavior Expert & Bestselling Author

INVISIBLE PAIN UNSTOPPABLE POWER

*A **PERSONAL JOURNEY** THROUGH BODY DYSMORPHIA, CHRONIC PAIN, AND **ENDOMETRIOSIS** THAT SPARKED A LIFE-CHANGING TRANSFORMATION*

KATYA KARLOVA

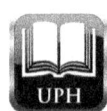

Invisible Pain Unstoppable Power
A Personal Journey Through Body Dysmorphia, Chronic Pain, and Endometriosis that Sparked a Life-Changing Transformation

Author: **Katya Karlova**
www.KatyaKarlova.com

Copyright © 2025 by Ultimate Publishing House
All rights reserved. No part of this book may be reproduced in any form or by any means without written permission from the publisher.

Attention: Permissions Coordinator
Ultimate Publishing House
205 Glen Shields Avenue
Toronto, Ontario, Canada
L4K 1T3
Email: info@ultimatepublishinghouse.com

Ultimate Publishing House – Bulk Orders & Corporate Gifting
Looking to elevate your brand or inspire your team? Bulk copies of Invisible Pain Unstoppable Power are available for companies, organizations, educational institutions, conferences, and client gifting.

Special Incentives for Bulk Orders:
✔ Orders of 100 copies or more qualify for special pricing.
✔ Orders of 1,000 copies or more receive deep volume discounts plus a complimentary custom second page featuring your logo, message from the CEO, or brand story — turning this book into a powerful branded asset or client gift.

Whether you're using it for leadership retreats, onboarding, holiday gifts, sponsorship bonuses, or brand awareness campaigns, this book becomes your voice in their hands.

To place a custom bulk order or to discuss tailored publishing solutions:
Call **Ultimate Publishing House**: 647-883-1758
www.ultimatepublishinghouse.com
Email: info@ultimatepublishinghouse.com

INVISIBLE PAIN UNSTOPPABLE POWER
AUTHOR KATYA KARLOVA
Transformative Leader. Resilience Coach. Speaker. Creator. Model.
ISBN: 979-8-9896573-6-0

DEDICATION

*To anyone and everyone on the invisible illness journey—
especially my fellow endo warriors—
This book is for you.*

*I know exactly how you're feeling. The dismissal. The
gaslighting. The medical trauma. The exhaustion. It's real.
And you are not alone.*

*I dedicate this book to all of you:
– Those currently suffering in silence
– Those waiting—often for years or decades—for a diagnosis
– And the incredible health professionals who have devoted
their lives to raising awareness, treating endometriosis and
other invisible illnesses, and tirelessly seeking not just a cure,
but real, lasting solutions.*

*My thoughts and prayers are with you—every day, every
hour, every minute.*

To those with endometriosis: we are called endo warriors because this is a battle. And it's only just beginning. But hear this clearly—we deserve better. And I believe, with everything in me, that one day we will rise as #EndoEmpresses—because this is not something we merely suffer from. It is something we live with.

No matter our struggle, we always have a choice in how we respond. And in that choice lies our power.

May this book be your roadmap. To healing. To strength. To turning invisible pain into unstoppable power.

FOREWORD

By Dr. John Demartini
*Human Behaviour Specialist, Visionary Teacher,
International Speaker, and Bestselling Author*

Every human being carries within them both visible stories and invisible struggles. Some of these struggles remain hidden for years, not because they are insignificant, but because society has not yet created the language—or the courage—to speak them aloud.

Katya Karlova's Invisible Pain, Unstoppable Power is a courageous unveiling of one such hidden journey. Through the lens of her experience with body dysmorphia, chronic pain, and endometriosis, she offers a profoundly honest narrative that transcends personal testimony and becomes a universal message of empowerment.

What struck me most while reading this book is how Katya transforms challenge into contribution. She does not position pain as a permanent prison, but rather as a teacher. She invites us to see beyond the suffering to the wisdom it contains. Pain, when embraced and understood, can become the very portal to power.

Her story demonstrates one of life's greatest paradoxes: that the very experiences which seem to break us open are the ones that give us access to our deepest strength. In the language of universal laws, opposites are always present. Where there is despair, there is hope. Where there is challenge, there is opportunity. Where there is pain, there is power.

Katya embodies this principle. She doesn't simply share her story—she transforms it into a roadmap for others who may still be in the shadows of their own battles. This book reminds us that every difficulty can serve as a stepping stone to greater resilience, greater purpose, and ultimately, greater service to humanity.

As you turn these pages, I invite you to not only witness Katya's journey, but to reflect on your own. Where have you mistaken obstacles for limitations, when they may in fact be openings? Where have you denied your own brilliance by focusing on the pain instead of the power?

Let this book be both a mirror and a catalyst. May it awaken within you the unstoppable force that already exists—waiting, quietly, behind whatever pain you carry.

With gratitude and admiration for Katya's contribution,

Dr. John Demartini

TABLE OF CONTENTS

FOREWORD vii
By Dr. John Demartini

Introduction
FACING THE INVISIBLE ENEMY 1

Chapter 1
BREAKING THE SILENCE – THE INVISIBLE
STRUGGLE 5

Chapter 2
THE CATALYST FOR CHANGE – HOW TRAUMA
SPARKED A TRANSFORMATION......................... 15

Chapter 3
FROM VICTIM TO EMPOWERED MINDSET............ 21

Chapter 4
THE POWER OF FEMININE ENERGY IN
TRANSFORMATION AND SUCCESS 37

Chapter 5
REWRITING THE SCRIPT — FROM VICTIMHOOD
TO EMPOWERED IDENTITY............................. 45

Chapter 6
ENERGETIC AUDIT – IDENTIFYING YOUR
CIRCLE'S IMPACT ON YOUR GROWTH 55

Chapter 7
THE CRUCIBLE OF QUIET: POWERING
THROUGH PRESENCE 65

Chapter 8
EMBODIED SELF-TRUST: LISTENING TO
YOUR INNER COMPASS 79

CHAPTER 9
THE TRUTH BENEATH THE PAIN:
RECLAIMING POWER THROUGH THE FEMININE 91

Chapter 10
THE SCIENCE OF SELF ADVOCACY 107

CHAPTER 11
FAITH, PURPOSE & THE SPIRITUAL PATH
TO HEALING... 121

Chapter 12
LIVING UNSTOPPABLE – INTEGRATING
POWER ACROSS EVERY ROLE 137

BONUS CHAPTERS
THE BOARDROOM QUEEN............................. 157

Endo-Friendly Anti-Inflammatory Nutrition Guide 165
GRATITUDE / NOTES 174
About The Author 183

ACKNOWLEDGEMENTS

Wow—where to begin?

I never imagined I would, or even could, write a book. But the fact that it was born out of necessity somehow makes it, I hope, all the more impactful. This work came from my own pain—so that others wouldn't have to feel as lost, dismissed, or alone as I did after my endometriosis diagnosis. And I couldn't have created it without the unwavering support of so many incredible people.

To everyone who encouraged me, mentored me, motivated me, held space for me, listened without judgment, wiped away tears, and pushed me to keep going—thank you. You know who you are, and I carry your love and strength with me every step of the way.

To my closest family and friends—you're private, and I respect that. But you've been my quiet pillars, and I'm endlessly grateful.

To my **mentor and book publisher, Felicia Pizzonia** — you've given me more than publishing guidance. You've taught me how to live in alignment, how to apply the law of attraction, how to lead with gratitude, and how to step into my highest self. Your wisdom, super creativity interwoven throughout my book and mentorship have changed the way I see the world—and myself. Thank you for encouraging me to reach for my wildest dreams and to teach others to do the same. Thank you to the entire Ultimate Publishing House team!

A special thank you to Tony Marinozzi, a fabulous connector whose support and introductions make a world of difference.

A heartfelt thank you to my dear friend **James Date**, who referred me to **Dr. Mollie Johnston** at UCLA, who then connected me with **Dr. Sheldon Jordan**. Dr. Jordan, your miraculous interventional pain techniques gave me a pathway to truly begin healing. I'm forever grateful.

To **Dr. Lyashevsky** at UCLA—you are the most caring, attentive, and knowledgeable primary care doctor I've ever encountered. You may not know it, but you likely saved my life. When I first met you, I was barely surviving—certainly not thriving—and your guidance helped me make the radical decision to put my health and myself first, for the very first time.

To **Dr. Andrea Vidali** at ESSI, thank you for your commitment, compassion, and care. You're not only an incredible physician, but a genuinely kind human being. And to **Dr. Sallie Sarrel**—

your advocacy and knowledge-sharing are leaving a lasting legacy that touches so many lives. I'm so grateful to know you. To the amazing women behind **@the_endo_space** on Instagram—thank you. For many of us, community pages like yours are the only place we find real understanding and trustworthy information. After years of dismissal, gaslighting, and shame, we turn to each other. Your work got me through some of my darkest days. Please never doubt the impact you're making.

To all the endo warriors, invisible illness fighters, and quiet heroes reading this—you've inspired every word. You are not alone. And this book is for you.

xoxo
Katya

INTRODUCTION
FACING THE INVISIBLE ENEMY

*"The only person you are destined to become
is the person you decide to be."*
— RALPH WALDO EMERSON

Invisible pain often feels like a silent enemy. It strikes without warning, leaves no physical scars, and yet it dominates the lives of those who face it. For many, this pain is invisible in the truest sense—whether it's the excruciating, unpredictable nature of chronic illness like endometriosis, the haunting thoughts tied to body dysmorphia, or the constant struggle with pain that others can't see, it can feel like a solitary battle. But what if the very fact that this pain is invisible is where the true power lies?

In *Invisible Pain, Unstoppable Power,* I invite you to walk with me through my journey of learning how to transform this silent pain into an unstoppable force. I have lived with conditions that seemed invisible to the world around me—conditions that wreaked havoc on my body and mind. I know firsthand how it feels to be misunderstood, to feel as though your struggles are invisible to everyone except you. Yet, over time, I discovered that it was through embracing this pain, through accepting it and facing it head-on, that I found my strength. My hope for this book is to help you do the same.

Endometriosis, chronic pain, body dysmorphia—these are not just conditions. They are life-changing battles, and they often leave us feeling powerless. But the truth is, we always have the power to choose how we respond to the challenges life hands us. This book is about giving you that power—tools for transforming your mindset, strategies for cultivating resilience, and a roadmap to discovering the strength within you that will carry you through the toughest times.

My goal is not to create another story of suffering but to offer you a blueprint for triumph—a reminder that no matter how dark the days may seem, the light is always within reach. You may feel weak, but within you lies an unstoppable power that, once awakened, will drive you forward, through pain and into purpose. As you read these pages, I encourage you to embrace the uncomfortable, to sit with the pain, and, most importantly, to rise from it stronger than ever before. Your journey to self-discovery and healing begins here. I was born in Moldova, a small country often overlooked on the map, yet filled with resilience, tradition, and simplicity. My childhood was shaped by a humble life — where neighbors leaned on each other, where gratitude was found in the little things, and where food

INTRODUCTION

came straight from the earth. Organic wasn't a label; it was our way of life. I can still remember the sweetness of fruit picked from our own trees, the richness of homemade bread, and the appreciation we held for every meal, every harvest, every shared moment.

Those early years gave me a foundation built on truth, health, and authenticity — values that would later guide me through some of the most challenging seasons of my life. As I grew, my path carried me far from the quiet gardens of Moldova into a world of modern complexity, where invisible struggles — chronic pain, body dysmorphia, and undiagnosed endometriosis — silently shaped my days.

What began as hidden suffering eventually became the catalyst for transformation. The lessons I carried from my roots — resilience, appreciation, and the belief that truth always finds its way to the surface — became the compass that guided me through the darkness. This book is born from that journey: a testimony that even in invisible pain, there is unstoppable power.

CHAPTER 1
BREAKING THE SILENCE – THE INVISIBLE STRUGGLE

"The most important decision you will ever make is to be in a good mood"
— Voltaire

I was thirteen when it first hit me. The pain—unbearable, crippling—was unlike anything I'd known. It wasn't a scrape from climbing trees or a bruise from tennis practice. It wasn't even the typical discomfort that comes with puberty. This was deep, unrelenting, and demanded my full attention. And though I didn't know it at the time, it marked the beginning of a decades-long battle with something invisible.

What started as a dull ache with my second period quickly spiraled into something much darker. It hit me in waves, like a storm tearing through my body from the inside. I couldn't stand. I couldn't think. I remember curling into a ball on the floor of my school's nurse's office, tears streaming down my face, clutching my abdomen, unsure if I would faint or vomit—or both. That was my introduction to a kind of pain that doesn't just exist in the body. It lodges itself into your psyche. It becomes a quiet, persistent companion.

At home, my mother tried everything. Heating pads. Ginger tea. Vicodin. It was a patchwork of home remedies and borrowed prescriptions. She was terrified but masked it with maternal calm. We didn't talk about illness in our home—not in a serious way. Pain was to be managed, endured, hidden. I was told, "It's just your period," and "Some girls have it worse than others." The message was clear: toughen up.

And so I did. Or at least, I tried.

THE GASLIGHTING BEGINS

Doctors told me I was overreacting. That I was too sensitive. That it was anxiety. Stress. Hormones. "You're just a teenager," one said with a smirk, as if being young invalidated my experience. Another doctor actually laughed when I asked if something might be wrong with me. I was handed birth control, anti-anxiety pills, even antidepressants. The message was loud and clear: It was all in my head.

It wasn't.

Endometriosis doesn't show up on blood tests or ultrasounds in the early stages. It hides in plain sight, disguising itself as "normal" menstrual pain. And because we live in a society that minimizes women's health issues—especially reproductive ones—many of us suffer in silence. I was no exception.

Years went by. I missed school, then work. I bailed on social events. I canceled dates. My friendships frayed. My identity began to erode. I wasn't the vibrant, athletic, high-achieving girl I used to be. I became "the flaky one," "the sick one," "the overly emotional one." I began to question everything about myself. Was I weak? Was I crazy? Was I broken?

THE COST OF SILENCE

The hardest part wasn't even the pain. It was the invisibility of it all. When you break your leg, people rush to sign your cast. When you have cancer, they bring casseroles. But when you have an invisible illness—especially one that revolves around periods and reproduction—people avert their eyes. They change the subject. They tell you to meditate more, stress less, eat better.

I started to internalize the silence. I stopped talking about my pain. I learned to mask it with makeup, with smiles, with fake laughs at parties when inside I was crumbling. I showed up to work with heating pads strapped under my clothes and bottles of painkillers in my purse. I learned how to dissociate—to leave my body during flareups just to get through the day.

But the cost was steep. Emotionally. Physically. Spiritually. The longer I stayed silent, the more I disappeared.

DIAGNOSIS AND THE BITTERSWEET TRUTH

It wasn't until my mid-thirties that I finally met a doctor who truly listened. For once, I wasn't dismissed with a shrug, a rushed prescription, or a vague suggestion that it was "all in my head." She leaned in. She asked thoughtful questions. She took careful notes. And then, almost quietly, she said a word I had never heard before: *endometriosis.*

I cried.

Not from fear. Not from devastation. I cried because someone finally believed me. After more than a decade of searching, the monster that had been living inside me had a name. My pain was real. It had always been real.

But the relief was fleeting. Endometriosis has no cure. There is no magic pill. What awaited me was a relentless cycle of surgeries, hormone treatments, dietary changes, and the exhausting task of trying to manage a disease that behaves like an unpredictable storm, striking without warning and leaving destruction in its wake

Over the years, I endured four surgeries—three of them performed by a surgeon I trusted, but who ultimately betrayed that trust. Her mistakes left permanent scars, not only across my abdomen but deep within the very fabric of my future. Each intervention chipped away at my hope, until the fourth one took everything. That surgery stole my uterus, my ability to carry children, and with it, an entire chapter of dreams I would never have the chance to write.

The grief was staggering. It came in waves—anger, disbelief, numbness, sorrow—each one heavier than the last. It wasn't just the loss of fertility. It was the loss of choices, of milestones, of the imagined life I had pictured since I was a girl.

Because endometriosis can only be definitively diagnosed through laparoscopic surgery, I had assumed that my surgeon was not only confirming the disease but treating it. Instead, I would later learn the truth: during my first three surgeries, she never removed the lesions at all. Whether it was ignorance, arrogance, or negligence, she left the disease to grow unchecked inside of me. By the time I underwent my hysterectomy—the fourth surgery in a single year—the video footage revealed what I had long suspected: the lesions had never been ablated or excised.

The consequences were irreversible. I had lost my uterus, my fertility, and was thrust into early menopause—not because of the disease alone, but because my first surgeon was not the expert she pretended to be.

SHIFTING FROM VICTIM TO WARRIOR

For a long time, I wore my diagnosis like a burden. A label. A limitation. But over time, something shifted. I realized that I couldn't control what was happening to my body—but I could control how I responded to it. That shift—from victim to warrior —was the most powerful transformation of my life.

It wasn't overnight. Healing never is. It took years of therapy, journaling, bodywork, and spiritual exploration. I had to rebuild my sense of self from the ground up. I had to re-learn how to trust my body. To love it. To thank it for surviving when I had treated it like the enemy.

I also began to connect with others who shared similar experiences. The community of women living with endometriosis, fibromyalgia, chronic fatigue, and other invisible illnesses became my lifeline. In them, I saw my own story reflected back at me. And I realized: I wasn't alone. I had never been alone.

FROM PAIN TO PURPOSE

One of the most radical things you can do in a world that silences your pain is to speak. Loudly. Clearly. With conviction. This book is my act of rebellion. My act of reclamation. It's my way of saying: I see you. I hear you. I believe you.

Your pain is real.
Your story matters.
And you are not broken.

You are becoming.

Every woman, every man, every non-binary person who has suffered in silence deserves a path to visibility, validation, and vitality. This book isn't just about endometriosis. It's about the alchemy of pain. It's about transforming trauma into power. It's about rewriting the story.

THE INVISIBLE BECOMES UNSTOPPABLE

As you journey through these chapters, I invite you to see yourself as the hero of your own story. You are not at the mercy of your body. You are not at the mercy of a broken medical system. You are powerful. You are intuitive. And you have the capacity to heal—not just physically, but emotionally and spiritually.

Let this be the moment where the silence ends.
Let this be the page where the power begins.

EXERCISE: RECLAIMING YOUR VOICE

This exercise is designed to help you break your own silence and begin the journey from invisible pain to unstoppable power.

STEP 1: VALIDATE YOUR EXPERIENCE

Write a letter to yourself as if you are your own best friend. Acknowledge what you've been through. Say everything you wish someone else had said to you. Be honest. Be kind. Be fierce.

STEP 2: REWRITE THE NARRATIVE

Answer the following:
- What has your pain taught you about yourself?
- What limiting beliefs have you held because of your diagnosis or condition?
- What new beliefs are you ready to adopt?

STEP 3: SPEAK IT OUT LOUD

Choose a safe space—your bedroom, a quiet walk in nature, or even a trusted friend—and read your letter aloud. Let your body hear your voice. Let your truth vibrate through your being.

CHAPTER 1

Repeat the following affirmation:
"My pain does not define me. My power is rising. I am no longer silent."

Welcome to your journey.
This is where the silence ends.
And where your unstoppable story begins.

Here is the full expanded version of ***Chapter 2: The Catalyst for Change – How Trauma Sparked a Transformation*** along with the 7 NLP-based exercises at the end:

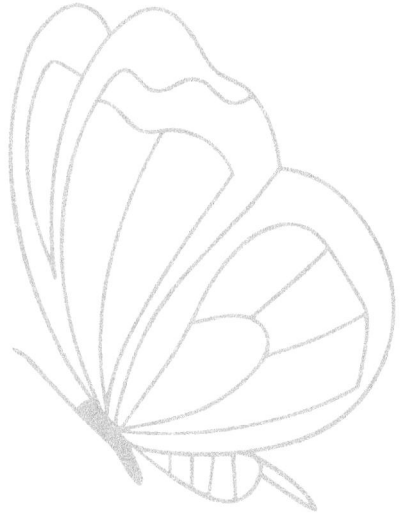

CHAPTER 2

THE CATALYST FOR CHANGE – HOW TRAUMA SPARKED A TRANSFORMATION

"Go confidently in the direction of your dreams, live the life you have imagined."
— HENRY DAVID THOREAU

There are moments in life that fracture us—but they also forge us. For years, I lived inside the paradox of pain and power. The trauma I endured—from the relentless cycles of undiagnosed endometriosis to the emotional exhaustion of not being believed—threatened to swallow me whole. But eventually, I stopped asking, "Why me?" and began asking, "What now?"

The moment we stop seeing ourselves as victims of circumstance and instead become authors of our own healing, we begin to awaken to a deeper truth: we are not broken—we are becoming.

At thirteen, I didn't have those words. I only had the visceral awareness of something being deeply wrong. The sharp, tearing agony that curled me into the fetal position wasn't just a rite of passage. It wasn't something "every girl goes through." It was something more sinister—and far more isolating.

Years of being gaslit, dismissed, and misdiagnosed followed. And yet, in the midst of that chaos, something quietly began to shift. I began to question the authority I once handed over so easily. I began to listen not just to the voices around me—but to the voice within.

The trauma didn't break me. It called me deeper. It beckoned me toward a kind of transformation no textbook or doctor could map out. It was the sacred unfolding of someone discovering that their pain had a purpose. That their body was not the enemy. That their voice, long silenced, carried the resonance of truth and resilience.

I began researching obsessively. Not out of fear, but out of a fierce desire to understand what was happening to me. And in that pursuit, I began healing—not just physically, but emotionally, mentally, spiritually. Healing was no longer a destination. It became an identity.

And here's the thing trauma taught me: pain is a truth-teller. It exposes what we ignore. It disrupts what no longer serves. It forces clarity. And in that brutal clarity, we discover our boundaries, our grit, and our power.

I came to see trauma not as a curse, but as a catalyst—a sacred ignition point that disrupted the status quo of my life and demanded something more from me. Something truer.

This wasn't about becoming perfect. It was about becoming whole.

And in that wholeness, I met women—and men—who had experienced their own catalytic pain. Divorce. Chronic illness. Abuse. Rejection. Miscarriage. Loss. What bound us together wasn't our wounds. It was our willingness to turn toward them and say: *You will not define me. You will refine me.*

Let this chapter remind you: you are not what happened to you. You are what you choose to become in response to it.

FINAL REFLECTION

What you've endured is not the end of you—it's the ignition point of something far more profound.

The weight you've carried, the silence you've survived, the ache that has shaped your days—none of it is meaningless. In fact, it's the raw material from which a stronger, more sovereign self is forged.

This isn't about silver linings or pretending the hurt didn't matter. It did. It does. But from that wreckage, something extraordinary can rise—not in spite of the pain, but because of how you faced it.

Let this not be the closing of your story, but the moment the real one begins.

NLP-BASED EXERCISES FOR INNER TRANSFORMATION

These 7 exercises are designed to help you reprogram your internal dialogue, regulate emotions, and step into your power using Neuro-Linguistic Programming techniques:

1. REFRAME THE MEANING

Write down a painful experience. Now list three empowering meanings it could hold in hindsight.

Examples:
What did it teach you? What strengths did it reveal?

2. FUTURE SELF VISUALIZATION

Close your eyes. Imagine the most empowered version of yourself one year from now. What are you wearing? How do you speak? What kind of people are around you? Step into that version. Journal what you see.

3. INTERRUPT THE PATTERN

Notice one repeating disempowering thought this week. When it surfaces, physically say:
"Cancel. That's not who I am anymore."

Then replace it with a new truth, e.g.,
"I am grounded, powerful, and wise."

4. CONFIDENCE ANCHOR

Recall a moment you felt proud, radiant, and strong. Stand tall. Press your thumb and middle finger together while breathing deeply into that state. Do this every morning to condition your nervous system.

5. REWRITE THE SCRIPT

Write 10 old beliefs that no longer serve you. Next to each one, write a new belief that uplifts and empowers you.

Say these aloud in front of a mirror each day for 21 days.

6. COLLAPSE THE EMOTION ANCHOR

When fear or sadness hits, shift your posture to a victory pose (arms up, open chest). Smile. Say an empowering phrase like:

"I am stronger than this."

This rewires your emotional response.

7. NLP GOAL ENCODING

Write one goal using this structure:
"I am **[positive action]** because I **[deep reason]**."

Example:
"I am sharing my story publicly because my truth inspires healing."

Read it daily with emotion and visualization.

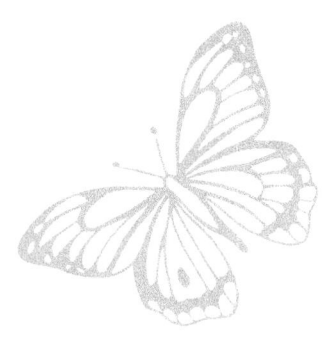

CHAPTER 3
FROM VICTIM TO EMPOWERED MINDSET

"Whether you think you can or think you can't you're right."
— HENRY FORD

Learning to transform a mindset of limitation into one of empowerment, and the steps to reclaim your personal power.

Shifting from a victim mindset to an empowered one is one of the most crucial transformations anyone can undergo. It is a fundamental realization that dictates how we navigate life's challenges. This shift is about recognizing the power we already hold within ourselves—the power to choose how we respond to circumstances.

A victim mindset is characterized by the belief that things are happening to us. It is a state of surrender to external forces, of feeling powerless in the face of adversity. But empowerment begins with the understanding that things are simply happening. They are not happening to us in a personal attack by the universe; they are just happening. And within that reality, we have the power to choose how we respond.

When faced with an obstacle, we must ask ourselves: Am I going to let this define me, or will I allow it to be just one chapter in my story? Am I merely surviving, or am I actively choosing to thrive?

This is not to say that hardships don't hurt or that the struggle isn't real. The pain can be overwhelming, and there will be moments where it feels unbearable. I recall a pivotal moment in my own journey—before my last major surgery, I was told I was severely anemic and needed immediate iron transfusions. I was already terrified of needles, and now I had to endure IVs in both arms. As I lay there, my initial thought was, Why is this happening to me? The weight of helplessness threatened to consume me. I started to feel the dizziness and tingling in my fingers that comes before a panic attack. It was as if my body knew before my mind could catch up that something was deeply wrong. The room tilted ever so slightly, sounds grew louder and sharper, and my chest tightened. I tried to steady my breath, to convince myself I was safe, but the spiral had already begun.

Then, a shift happened. This is not happening to me, I reminded myself. This is simply something that is happening. I had a choice: I could resist, panic, and spiral deeper into frustration, or I could accept the circumstances and make the best of them. So instead of sinking into misery, I chose to chat with the nurses, to make friends, to find laughter in the moment. That decision made all the difference.

Shift happens when we embrace that reality. Life is unpredictable, and adversity is inevitable. But whether we allow these experiences to shatter us or strengthen us is up to us. Nothing is in the way; it is on the way.

BREAKING FREE FROM THE MIND'S PRISON

One of the greatest barriers to empowerment is ourselves. Over the course of our lives, we develop a narrative—a story we tell ourselves about who we are and what we are capable of. Too often, that narrative is tainted with self-doubt, fear, and limitations. It's as if we are running on a default program, one rooted in negativity and limiting beliefs.

But here's the question to ask yourself: Is the way I currently think serving me? If not, then it's time for a change. Let's be real—sometimes the most dangerous place we can be is alone with our thoughts when those thoughts haven't been vetted for truth.

Many people become paralyzed by the fear of failure. They engage in endless analysis, predicting every possible negative outcome, and ultimately, they take no action. They let the fear of what if prevent them from taking that first step. But here's a radical idea: What if it works? What if everything turns out better than you could have imagined? What if the thing you're avoiding is the very gateway to everything you want?

There's something powerfully ironic about fear: it's often just poorly rehearsed faith in the wrong direction. Flip the script. Become your own inner hype-person.

CHOOSING EMPOWERMENT OVER FEAR

Empowerment requires accountability, and accountability is uncomfortable. Many people resist change because it means acknowledging that they are responsible for their own lives. That's a daunting realization. But it's also liberating—because if you have the power to change your mindset, you have the power to change your life.

Faith plays a huge role in this transformation. Whether you believe in the universe, a higher power, or simply the miraculous architecture of cause and effect, having faith that things are happening for a reason allows you to trust the process. It doesn't mean sitting back and waiting for miracles. It means aligning your actions with your vision.

Here's a cosmic truth bomb: Life doesn't reward the most deserving. It rewards the most aligned. Are your thoughts, words, actions, and environment aligned with the empowered life you say you want?

THE ROLE OF GRATITUDE IN HEALING

Gratitude is not spiritual fluff. It's strategic power. In every moment, we are tuning the radio of our minds. Tune into bitterness and you'll get static. Tune into gratitude, and you amplify clarity.

During my most difficult moments, I learned to practice gratitude for my body instead of resenting it. My body has carried me through so much. Instead of battling it, I learned to support it, to nourish it, to love it. That mental shift—going from "my body is broken" to "my body is fighting for me"—changed everything.

Radical gratitude is the skill of thanking the chaos for making you the conductor. It's when you can look back at your lowest point and say, "Ah, so that's why the fire had to burn."

RECOGNIZING THE UNIVERSE'S MESSAGES

Call it divine timing, synchronicity, serendipity—or just really good intuition with sneakers on. The universe is always speaking, and spoiler alert: it doesn't always use words.

One of the most sacred moments I experienced came through something as delicate as a butterfly. During the pandemic lockdown, I found solace in my garden; there was something about watching life push through the soil that brought me joy. On one trip to the nursery, a brilliant orange-flowered bush caught my eye, and I brought it home—unaware that it was milkweed, the very plant monarch butterflies choose as their nursery. And the next was nothing short of incredible! Within weeks, I began to notice delicate monarch butterflies circling the garden, landing on the very milkweed I had unknowingly planted for them. What started as a simple impulse purchase had become a sanctuary, a place where transformation was unfolding right before my eyes.I was planting milkweed without knowing it was the monarch's nursery of choice. I had no idea I was laying the groundwork for transformation—both theirs and mine. What followed was a front-row seat to one of nature's most miraculous metamorphoses. Caterpillars became cocoons. Cocoons became wings.

And me? I became someone who believed in my own rebirth. That was no coincidence. That was a spiritual mic drop.

LIVING IN ALIGNMENT WITH YOUR PURPOSE

Purpose isn't a to-do list—it's a to-be list. Who are you becoming as you go through this life? Not just what are you doing?

You know you're on the right path when you feel energy instead of fatigue. When your soul whispers "more of this" instead of "get me out of here."

I once worked in a space that was all deadlines and no lifelines. I was praised, promoted—and completely unfulfilled. That's when I realized: comfort zones are pretty, but nothing ever blooms there.

Your purpose is often disguised as your passion's most persistent whisper. The thing you keep pushing away, that keeps coming back stronger. Spoiler alert: that's not coincidence. That's divine persistence.

We are not here to simply exist. We are here to dance with life, not tiptoe around it. To lean in, to rise up, and to own our stories in every chapter.

SHIFT HAPPENS. AND WHEN IT DOES, IT CHANGES EVERYTHING.

Embrace it all and understand that nothing is good or bad, it is all perception. Your current "problem" might be your future punchline or your most powerful proof.

Don't view something in a negative light but understand it is there to serve you and act as a stepping stone to massive growth.

You're not broken—you're breaking open.
You're not behind—you're being prepared.

And you're definitely not powerless. You, my friend, are potent beyond belief.
Now, go claim it.

EXPANDED EMPOWERMENT INTEGRATION EXERCISES: UNLOCKING YOUR PERSONAL POWER

Empowerment is not just an idea—it's a practice. Like a muscle, your empowered mindset needs regular engagement. Below is a series of dynamic, multi-generational exercises that blend NLP (Neuro-Linguistic Programming), quantum principles, and emotional intelligence techniques to support you in embodying your transformation.

These practices are tailored for all walks of life—whether you're a student navigating identity, a working parent juggling roles, a creative carving a path, or a professional reclaiming joy. Start with what resonates most and trust the rest will meet you when you're ready.

1. THE NARRATIVE FLIP: REWRITE THE STORY YOU TELL YOURSELF

Who it's for:
Everyone, especially those feeling stuck or misjudged by past experiences.

- Write down a recurring negative thought or internal script you hear often (e.g., "I'm too much" or "No one listens to me").

- Flip it using evidence from your life. What's the opposite? (e.g., "I bring vibrant energy that ignites change." or "My voice has created impact and comfort.")

- Place this rewritten truth somewhere visible—a mirror, journal, phone screen.

Why it works:
Rewiring language reframes your identity, which reframes your outcomes.

2. QUANTUM LEAP VISUALIZATION

Who it's for:
Entrepreneurs, dreamers, those at a crossroads.

- Close your eyes. Imagine yourself one year into the future living as your most empowered self.

- Observe the details: How do you walk into a room? How do others greet you? What are you wearing? What energy do you project?

- Anchor this version of you with a physical gesture—a hand on your heart or fist raised.

- Commit to embodying one habit of this future self starting today.

Bonus:
Name this future version of yourself and refer to them when making bold decisions.

3. THE MIRROR METHOD: IDENTITY UPGRADING

Who it's for:
Teens, creatives, and anyone with low self-esteem or body image struggle.

- Every morning and night, look into your eyes in the mirror and say aloud:
  - "I see you."
  - "I love you."
  - "I forgive you."
  - "I empower you."

- Add your own affirmations like "I am becoming who I was always meant to be."

Why it works:
Direct eye contact with yourself strengthens self-recognition, rewires shame, and restores confidence.

4. LEGACY LETTER EXERCISE

Who it's for:
Parents, professionals, caregivers, elders.

- Write a letter to your future grandchildren, mentees, or next-generation leaders.

- Share a truth you've learned from pain.

- Share what courage looked like for you when no one else saw.

- Close it with what you hope the next generation will embody.

Why it works:
Legacy reframes adversity into service. Your story becomes someone else's survival guide.

5. EMOTION TRANSMUTATION RITUAL

Who it's for:
Anyone healing grief, heartbreak, or betrayal.

- Identify a lingering emotion (anger, fear, regret).

- Set a timer for 10 minutes and free-write everything about that emotion. Do not edit.

- Safely burn or tear the paper while repeating:
  - "This emotion is energy. I choose to reclaim it as power."

- Close your eyes, breathe deeply, and place both hands over your heart.

Why it works:
This quantum-inspired ritual transforms stuck energy into intentional, embodied release.

6. GRATITUDE TIME-TRAVEL

Who it's for:
Anyone looking to fall back in love with life.

- Write a thank-you note to a future version of yourself 5 years from now.

- Thank them for healing. For choosing the hard path. For thriving against all odds.

- Let the note become your new north star. Revisit when you feel lost.

Pro Tip:
Record yourself reading it with music and listen when you wake up.

7. EMPOWERMENT PLAYLIST (GENERATIONAL VIBE LIFT)

Who it's for:
Everyone! But especially Gen Z, Gen Alpha, and Millennials.

- Create a playlist called "Empowered Me." Add:
  - Songs that remind you of triumph.
  - Songs you danced to as a kid.
  - Songs that make you feel like a hero or warrior.

- Play it before interviews, workouts, or when imposter syndrome creeps in.

Why it works:
Sound frequencies affect your emotional and mental state—use music as medicine.

8. ENERGY AUDIT: WHO GETS YOUR POWER?

Who it's for:
Empaths, people-pleasers, and those setting boundaries.

- List the five people you spend the most time thinking about or giving energy to.

- Next to each name, rate from 1–10 how they impact your emotional health.

- Circle anyone under 5. Reflect: What boundaries or conversations need to happen?

DAILY EMPOWERMENT PROMPTS

Use these prompts each morning or night to integrate the chapter's core ideas:

- What did I reclaim today?

- Where did I choose love over fear?

- What am I grateful for in this very moment?

- What would my empowered self do next?

CLOSING THOUGHT:

You are not here to live in reaction. You are here to respond—with power, with grace, with vision.

> *"You are not a drop in the ocean.*
> *You are the entire ocean in a drop."*
> — RUMI

Welcome to your new identity: not a victim of life, but a creator within it.

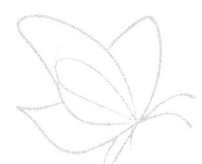

NOW ASK YOURSELF:

What would change today if you truly believed that you are enough—right here, right now?

CHAPTER 4

THE POWER OF FEMININE ENERGY IN TRANSFORMATION AND SUCCESS

"Courage is resistance to fear, mastery of fear, not absence of fear."
— MARK TWAIN

REFRAMING REJECTION: FROM DOUBT TO MAGNETIC POWER

Rejection is an unavoidable part of life. It's something everyone experiences, and yet, it holds so many people back. The fear of rejection paralyzes potential, but the truth is, rejection isn't a sign of failure—it's redirection. What is meant for you will find you. If something doesn't work out, it simply wasn't aligned with your journey.

The key to transforming rejection into magnetic power lies in embracing feminine energy. While masculine energy is about pursuing and pushing forward, feminine energy is about *being*—being open, receptive, and aligned. Women often feel the need to chase, to force outcomes, to prove their worth. But true feminine power lies in knowing that what is meant for you will naturally gravitate toward you.

The same principle applies to relationships. A woman who embodies her authenticity and confidence will naturally attract the right people into her life—whether in love, friendships, or business. The lesson? *Don't chase. Align.*

BALANCING THE MASCULINE AND FEMININE IN RELATIONSHIPS

There is a common misconception that equality means sameness. True balance in relationships comes from recognizing and honoring the differences between masculine and feminine energies. Masculine energy is goal-oriented, driven, and assertive, while feminine energy is intuitive, nurturing, and receptive. Both are powerful. One is not superior to the other.

A man who is truly in his masculine energy *wants* to pursue, to court, to provide. When a woman embraces her feminine energy, she allows space for the masculine energy to lead without resistance, not out of weakness, but out of confidence in her own value. It's not about submission—it's about *synergy*. True feminine power is not about control; it's about influence.

HOW WOMEN UNKNOWINGLY SABOTAGE INTIMACY

One of the biggest ways women self-sabotage intimacy is by assuming men think and process emotions the same way they do. Women often project their own thoughts, fears, and insecurities onto their partners, interpreting neutral situations through the lens of past wounds.

This unconscious projection leads to unnecessary conflicts and misunderstandings. The key to breaking this cycle is self-awareness. Before reacting, ask: *Is this feeling based on fact, or am I projecting an old story onto this situation?*

Healthy intimacy starts with emotional intelligence. Knowing yourself, your triggers, and your patterns allows you to engage in relationships with clarity rather than from a place of past hurt.

THE LINK BETWEEN FEMININE ENERGY AND ABUNDANCE

A woman's ability to receive love, money, and opportunities is directly tied to her ability to embrace her feminine energy. Feminine energy is receptive—it's about allowing, not forcing. Many women struggle with receiving because they don't believe they are *worthy* of what they desire.

This internal conflict creates *incongruence*—you say you want abundance, but internally, you resist it. The universe responds to vibration, not just words. If deep down you believe you're unworthy of success, love, or happiness, you will unconsciously repel it.

The solution? *Do the work.* Heal the wounds that tell you you're not enough. Step into your power. Allow abundance to come to you instead of chasing it from a place of lack.

FEMININE ENERGY IN BUSINESS AND LEADERSHIP

For years, business success was defined by traditionally masculine traits—logic, decisiveness, competition. But the rise of emotional intelligence in leadership has proven that feminine energy is just as crucial.

Empathy, intuition, collaboration, creativity—these are all feminine qualities that make for exceptional leadership. A truly powerful leader, regardless of gender, balances both energies.

In high-stakes negotiations, feminine energy creates a strategic advantage. Where two competing masculine energies might butt heads, a leader who leans into emotional intelligence can diffuse conflict, foster connection, and drive win-win outcomes.

THE DANGER OF OVERCOMPENSATING IN RELATIONSHIPS

Many women unknowingly push love away by overcompensating. They give too much, invest too much, and expect that their effort will earn them love. But love isn't a transaction.

Overcompensating often stems from fear—the fear of abandonment, of not being good enough, of being left behind. But this fear-based energy repels rather than attracts. Instead of proving your worth through excessive effort, step into your confidence. Trust that you are enough, exactly as you are. *Energy doesn't lie—operate from love, not fear.*

THE IMPACT OF SUPPRESSED EMOTIONS ON RELATIONSHIPS

When women suppress emotions, they create inner turmoil that inevitably affects their relationships. Unspoken resentments build, leading to passive-aggressiveness, emotional outbursts, or complete disengagement.

Instead of bottling up emotions, practice *self-reflection* and *conscious communication*. Address issues as they arise, with clarity and honesty, before they turn into toxic patterns.

A WOMAN'S RELATIONSHIP WITH HER FATHER AND ITS EFFECT ON LOVE & SUCCESS

A woman's early relationship with masculine energy—often represented by her father—plays a crucial role in her love life and professional success. If a father was absent, controlling, or emotionally unavailable, a woman may develop unresolved wounds that manifest in her adult relationships.

However, childhood experiences do not dictate destiny. *Healing is a choice.* Regardless of the past, every woman has the power to redefine her relationship with masculine energy—whether in men, money, or power. The key is *resolution*. When past wounds are acknowledged and healed, they no longer shape future relationships.

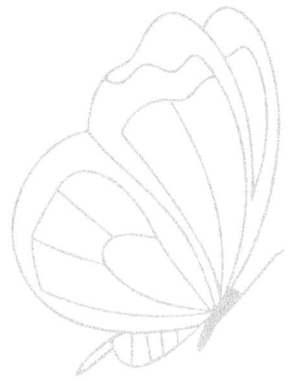
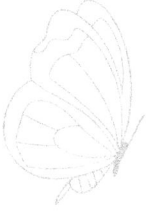

CHAPTER 4

EXERCISE: RECLAIMING YOUR FEMININE POWER

Take some time to complete this guided exercise to align with your feminine energy and open yourself to receiving abundance in all areas of life.

1. **Reflection:**
   Find a quiet space and journal about your relationship with receiving. Do you allow yourself to receive love, support, compliments, or financial abundance freely? Or do you feel guilt, fear, or unworthiness?

2. **Identify Blocks:**
   Write down any limiting beliefs you have around femininity, relationships, success, and abundance. Where did these beliefs come from? Are they yours, or were they passed down to you?

3. **Affirmations:**
   Create affirmations that counter those limiting beliefs. Some examples:
   - *I am worthy of love and abundance.*
   - *I receive with grace and gratitude.*
   - *I am in perfect balance with my feminine and masculine energy.*

4. **Practice Receiving:**
   For one week, make a conscious effort to receive without resistance. Accept compliments without deflecting. Allow others to support you without feeling the need to give back immediately. Observe how this shifts your energy.

5. **Visualization:**
   Close your eyes and visualize yourself embodying your feminine power. See yourself moving with ease, attracting opportunities, and being in a space of full confidence and grace.

FINAL THOUGHT:

Nothing is inherently good or bad—it is our *perception* that gives it meaning. When you shift your perspective, you shift your reality. Challenges aren't obstacles; they are opportunities for growth.

Embrace it all. Recognize that every experience—pain, joy, love, loss—is serving you in some way. Step into your feminine power, not as a means to control, but as a way to align with your highest self. The world is waiting for you to step into your full potential. Be ready to receive.

CHAPTER 5

REWRITING THE SCRIPT — FROM VICTIMHOOD TO EMPOWERED IDENTITY

"The first wealth is health."
— Ralph Waldo Emerson

INTRODUCTION: WHAT IF YOU'RE NOT BROKEN?

We live in a culture that loves to diagnose and define. Pain becomes pathology. Struggle becomes identity. Labels like "chronic," "invisible," or "disorder" become part of how we see ourselves. But what if you were never broken to begin with?

This chapter is about more than mindset—it's about radical reclamation. It's the pivot point where invisible pain becomes visible strength. Where the story shifts from "Why me?" to "Watch me."

INVISIBLE ILLNESS AND EMOTIONAL IDENTITY

Most people assume invisible pain refers only to physical ailments—autoimmune disease, fibromyalgia, endometriosis. But its shadow stretches further. There's the emotional pain of not being believed, the psychological ache of internalized shame, and the existential fatigue of asking, "Will anyone ever really see me?"

Women and men alike carry silent burdens. For many, pain became a defining narrative early in life. Childhood neglect. Abuse. A dysfunctional relationship with our body. Over time, we began to *expect* pain. We braced for it. We stopped demanding more.

"When pain becomes familiar, joy can feel suspicious."

But here's the truth: your pain is not your fault. But your power? That *is* your responsibility.

THE MINDSET SHIFT: RESPONSE OVER REACTION

Victimhood is reactive. Empowerment is responsive. The difference? Ownership.

I share a pivotal moment in my healing journey—being turned away from surgery due to anemia. Hooked up to two IVs, terrified of needles, in a clinic surrounded by cancer patients, I could've spiraled into despair. But I didn't.

I made a choice: "I'm here. This is happening. And I can either suffer *through* it or rise *within* it."

I made jokes with the nurses. I laughed through the discomfort. I made the unbearable... bearable.

This was not spiritual bypassing. This was *transmutation*—the art of choosing presence over panic.

SELF-PERCEPTION: THE ORIGINAL NARRATIVE

Most people have never questioned the internal narrative running on repeat since childhood.
- "I'm not enough."
- "Nothing ever works out for me."
- "My body is betraying me."

But what if that voice wasn't *yours* to begin with? What if that story was inherited—from culture, trauma, or well-meaning but wounded caregivers?

Reclaiming your power starts with rewriting your self-concept. Not with delusion, but with deep intention.

"I am not the voice in my head. I am the one listening—and choosing a new script."

THE POWER OF NAMING

To heal, you have to *name* what's been buried. Not for the world's validation—but for your own.
- Name the betrayal.
- Name the diagnosis.
- Name the disappointment.

Naming doesn't mean obsessing. It means witnessing. And only what's witnessed can be transformed.

SHIFTING IDENTITY: FROM ILLNESS TO INSIGHT

There comes a moment in every healing journey when you stop asking, "How do I fix myself?" and start asking, "How do I support who I am now?"

This is where true healing begins.

I share how chronic illness forced me to release the identity of perfectionism. No more chasing the perfect body. The perfect job. The perfectly curated life. Instead, I learned to *receive*—support, rest, gentleness, truth.

> *"You don't heal by becoming who you were.
> You heal by becoming who you actually are."*

THE ROLE OF SOMATICS AND SELF-AWARENESS

The body holds the story long after the mind has moved on. That's why affirmations aren't enough. The nervous system must feel safe to shift.

Somatic tools like:
- Gentle breathwork
- Body scans
- Mirror work
- Movement with emotional intention

…are critical. Healing isn't just mental—it's cellular.

Each time you lovingly place your hand on your belly and say, "I've got you," you rewire decades of abandonment.

Each time you choose rest over productivity, you say: "My worth is not measured in output."

CASE STUDY: FROM COLLAPSE TO COMMAND

Meet Devon—a 39-year-old father of two. For years, he silently battled fibromyalgia and depression. On the outside, he was high-performing. Inside, he was imploding.

After reading my book, something clicked. For the first time, he acknowledged: "I'm not lazy. I'm in pain. And I deserve help."

He started journaling daily. He joined a men's trauma group. He stopped numbing. He started *feeling*.

Today, Devon still has hard days. But he's no longer drowning in secrecy. He's a present father. A vulnerable leader. An empowered man.

> *"When you own your pain, you own your power.*
> *One breath at a time."*

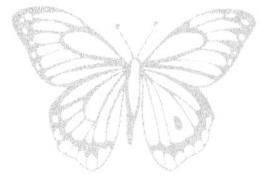

DAILY PRACTICES TO ANCHOR A NEW IDENTITY

1. **Morning Alignment Check**

   Ask: "What version of me is leading today—my past or my potential?"
   Adjust accordingly.

2. **Radical Reframing**

   Every time you think "I can't," add: "...yet."
   Every time you catch yourself spiraling, say: "I'm choosing a new path."

3. **Nourishment Before Achievement**

   Replace the to-do list with a "to-feel" list.
   What would make you feel supported today?

REAL TALK ON FEAR AND RESISTANCE

Resistance isn't laziness—it's self-protection. Your brain is trying to keep you alive, not help you thrive. But safety doesn't live in old patterns.

Safety lives in the *present*. In truth-telling. In allowing discomfort without labeling it as danger.

"Your nervous system doesn't need to be fixed. It needs to be heard."

INTEGRATION EXERCISES

Rewrite the Pain Narrative

- Write a letter to your younger self, validating everything they felt.
- Then write a response from your current self, showing how far you've come.

Mirror Ritual

Stand in front of a mirror for 3 minutes. Say aloud:
- I am not broken.
- My body is my ally.
- I am healing.

Future Self Visualization

Close your eyes. Picture your healthiest, most radiant self. Ask them:
- What do I need to let go of?
- What am I ready to receive?

CHAPTER 5

FINAL REFLECTION

The most radical thing you can do is choose not to abandon yourself. Again. Especially when the pain is loud, when the world is overwhelming, or when your inner critic is screaming the loudest. In those moments, choose yourself again and again. This is not about ignoring what hurts — it's about facing it with love, grace, and grit.

You are not just recovering from pain. You are becoming someone new. Someone refined by fire, softened by wisdom, and emboldened by choice. Every breath you take is evidence of your resilience. Every time you choose rest over pushing, compassion over criticism, or truth over performance — you are rewriting the very foundation of your life.

Someone who owns their truth. Someone who embodies resilience. Someone who can hold the weight of the past with the lightness of compassion.

You are not here to stay small. You are not here to be defined by what went wrong. You are here to transform pain into purpose, survival into sovereignty, and silence into strength. Let this chapter — and this moment — be the beginning of a new way of seeing yourself: not as someone who barely got through it, but as someone who rose with grace, fire, and the wisdom to guide others.

This is your time. This is your turning point. Your story is far from over. In fact — it's just beginning.

Step forward now. Unapologetically.
Unstoppably. Fully YOU.

You are not broken. You are becoming.

You are not your pain. You are your power.

You are unstoppable.

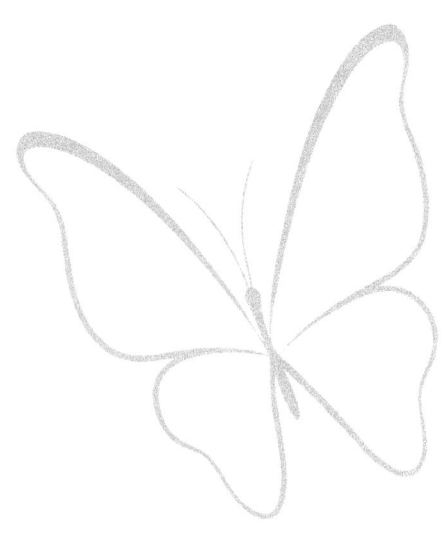

CHAPTER 6

ENERGETIC AUDIT – IDENTIFYING YOUR CIRCLE'S IMPACT ON YOUR GROWTH

"Let food be thy medicine and medicine be thy food."
— HIPPOCRATES

We often hear the phrase, *you are the sum of the five people you spend the most time with.* But have you ever taken a moment to truly evaluate who is in your inner circle and how they contribute to your personal growth? The truth is, relationships are not just about history, proximity, or even shared experiences; they are about alignment and energy. Who we allow into our personal space—emotionally, mentally, and physically—deeply affects our success, mindset, and overall well-being.

Gossip, complaining, and negativity are some of the lowest vibrational frequencies that can cloud your energy and dim your potential. If you consistently find yourself surrounded by people who gossip, dwell in negativity, or project their fears onto you, it may be time to reevaluate their role in your life. While it can feel difficult—especially when it involves long-term friendships or family members—the most liberating realization is this: **you are not obligated to maintain relationships that keep you from stepping into your highest self**.

Many people resist making necessary changes because of one underlying fear—loneliness. *If I let go of these friendships, who will I have left?* But the real question is: *If you continue to surround yourself with people who don't align with your growth, who will you become?* True transformation requires pruning—the same way a gardener trims away dead leaves to allow new life to flourish.

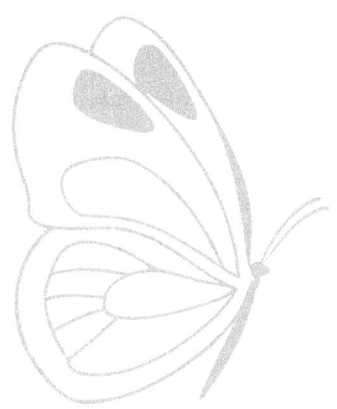

CHAPTER 6

THE ENERGETIC AUDIT: WHO'S SUPPORTING VS. WHO'S STUNTING YOUR SUCCESS?

STEP 1:
REFLECT ON YOUR CORE CIRCLE

Write down the names of the five people you interact with the most in your daily life. These can be friends, colleagues, family members, or even mentors. Be honest and include the people who consume the majority of your time and energy.

Name: --

Name: --

Name: --

Name: --

Name: --

Name: --

STEP 2:
IDENTIFY THEIR IMPACT

For each person, ask yourself the following questions:
- Do I feel **energized** or **drained** after spending time with this person?
- Do they encourage my **growth** or reinforce my **old patterns**?
- Are they **contributing** to my well-being and success, or are they **consuming** my energy?
- Do they offer **constructive support** or **subtle competition**?
- When I share my dreams, do they **support** or **sabotage** them?
- Do they elevate my **mindset** or feed my **self-doubt**?

Write down your reflections:

Person 1:

Person 2:

Person 3:

Person 4:

Person 5:

STEP 3:
CATEGORIZE YOUR CIRCLE

Using your answers, categorize the people in your life into three groups:

- **Contributors:**
  These individuals support your vision, encourage you, and bring positive energy into your life.

- **Neutral:**
  These relationships don't particularly lift you up, but they don't weigh you down either.

- **Consumers:**
  These people drain your energy, distract you from your goals, or reinforce limiting beliefs.

Write down the names of each category:

Contributors:

Neutral:

Consumers:

STEP 4:
MAKE ADJUSTMENTS

Now, take action based on what you've discovered:

- **Increase time with Contributors:**
  Find ways to deepen your connection with those who uplift and inspire you.

- **Set boundaries with Neutrals:**
  Limit time with those who don't add value but don't necessarily harm you.

- **Gracefully distance from Consumers:**
  Reduce or eliminate interactions with those who hold you back, and do so with love and detachment.

Action Plan:

STEP 5:
CREATE AN ENERGETIC INTENTIONS LIST

Write down 3-5 traits you want in the people who surround you. Examples:

- Encourages my dreams
- Challenges me to be my best self
- Celebrates my success without jealousy
- Brings positivity and high energy
- Engages in meaningful, growth-oriented conversations

Your Ideal Traits:

Whenever you meet new people, evaluate them against this list before fully integrating them into your inner circle.

FINAL THOUGHT: ELEVATE TO ALIGN

Your future self depends on the people you surround yourself with today. As you elevate, you will naturally align with people who match your energy. Let go of the fear of loneliness—because in that space, you are making room for the high-caliber connections that are truly meant to be part of your journey.

Are you ready to step into your highest vibration?

Complete this audit and take control of the energy in your life. You deserve a circle that reflects your growth, power, and unstoppable potential.

Notes & Reflections:

NOTES

CHAPTER 7

THE CRUCIBLE OF QUIET: POWERING THROUGH PRESENCE

"The secret to getting ahead is getting started."
— Mark Twain

I still felt the sting of that email late that morning, when the rain drizzled on my windowsill and the kettle's final whistle echoed behind me. The screen lit up with the words no one wants to read: *"We regret to inform you..."* Dressed up in polished HR language, the message was unmistakable—I didn't get the job.

Just like that, the world narrowed. My coffee grew cold, as if in solidarity with the collapse in my chest. The momentum of my day—my life—pressed forward, but I felt stuck inside a crater of doubt.

That's the paradox of rejection: it lands like a blow, yet it demands we look within. With trembling fingertips, I closed the laptop and sat in silence. My body rattled with adrenaline, grief, shame—a cocktail I'd been numbing for years with busyness, hustle, productivity. Not today. Today, I refused to escape. Today, I invited the fracture.

I paced across my living room in slow arcs, following the current of my breath. Each inhale brought in vulnerability; each exhale carried a word: "This pain… is not failure." I let tears come, even before I allowed the thought. It felt messy. It felt dangerous. It felt alive.

And through the haze of self-judgment, I heard a question: *What if this moment isn't an end, but a catalyst?* That whisper didn't fix me. It simply reminded me I still breathed. That I still could reclaim my own locus of meaning.

I found my favorite journal and wrote just one line: "*I am sacred. I am enough.*"

And then I paused. Something cracked open. Not because I wanted it to—but because I needed it to.

For days, I lit a candle each morning and allowed myself to sit quietly, surrendering to emptiness rather than rushing to fill it. I got curious about how it felt to linger in a space devoid of solutions. I noticed my throat tended to tighten when I spoke about setbacks; my chest clenched whenever I thought I had to fix everything right away.

In those patrols of my own body, I discovered patterns I'd never witnessed. I realized how much of my identity was tied to achievements and external validation. The small 12-worthiness part of me—parental praise, corporate titles, social currency—still flinched at loss. Still asked for ladders and metrics. It was all still there, consuming neural energy, shaping my sense of permission.

But deeper than the chase, under the habit loops, I found something more fundamental. A pulse of resonance—a quiet aliveness that didn't need explanation or outcome. I didn't name it "confidence" or "power." I called it "presence."

Presence didn't have to perform. It didn't have to secure. It simply *was*. It invited a deeper type of potency—a power that didn't roar but grounded everything it touched.

In the following weeks, I experimented with this idea in micro ways:

I showed up for a tough video call. Before diving in, I closed my eyes for 30 seconds, hands on my heart, and breathed deeply into my chest. During the meeting, I spoke less and tuned more—watching, noticing shifts in energy. My contributions emerged from a quieter place, but carried more weight.

In conversation with my partner, instead of "You're wrong, hear me," I said: *"I feel tension. I'm wondering what's alive between us."* Silence followed. Then speech that felt more generative than defensive.

At dinner with friends, I dropped the default "how am I doing?" performance script—no brag, no stumble—just softness and receptivity. And people leaned in. They shared deeper parts of themselves. They were mirroring back that I didn't need fixes—I could just *be*.

The irony was undeniable: less chasing created more connection. Less showing up strong created more invitation. Less hurry created more impact.

This is the alchemy Murdock describes in the Heroine's Journey: the descent, the shadow, the integration. It's not about taking away pain—it's about refining into wholeness. It's about letting the current of your own nervous system become your compass.

I began each day with a small ritual:

1. **Meditation for 5 minutes.**
   Sitting upright, eyes closed, palms open. I labeled thoughts "thinking" and returned to breath. Rooted in the sound of my own breath, I anchored into presence.

2. **Sensation check.**

    I scanned my body—jaw, chest, belly—held space for what was present. If I felt tightness, I breathed into it. If I felt release, I allowed it to expand.

3. **Word of the day.**

    One word—*softness, grounded, clarity*—that anchored intention.

4. **Evening reflection.**

    I wrote one sentence about how presence showed up in my day.

I need to tell you about my father. His presence in my life was foundational yet startlingly brief. He provided for our family, traveled constantly, and returned wearing exhaustion. His love was sure, but his availability was not. I grew up learning that love is earned, and to earn required action. It shaped my internal script: do more, prove worth, chase approval.

Writing a letter to him was one of the most disarming acts I've ever done. There was no expectation that he'd read it. The letter began with gratitude—for the lessons, the care, the sacrifices. Then I spoke of absence—not to indict, but to acknowledge. *"I forgive you—and I forgive me for building my worth outside myself."* I wrote until tears blurred my ink. Then I closed it and burned it in my backyard under rising stars.

Since then, I haven't needed permission to show up as I am. I anchor to presence—not to performance.

The next challenge: rejection at work. I whispered to myself before turning my camera on: *I belong here, even in this disappointment.* I watched my colleagues' jaws soften. I watched someone sit up straighter after I spoke my truth—not as someone trying to shine, but as someone rooted in self.

By the end of the quarter, the director gave me a nod: "I appreciate the presence you bring. You shifted the energy in this project." And yes—that felt good. But more than those words, it was the recognition that *I didn't need them* to feel enough. I had brought enough by simply being.

You may ask: "But what about accomplishments? What about results?" I'm not saying those don't matter. They do. But what I'm suggesting is that chasing them from a place of emptiness—seeking them to validate our worth—is a weakening posture. When we can not only produce results—but also *embody calm, firmness, generosity*, regardless of outcomes... we become unstoppable.

Presence doesn't guarantee comfort. Sometimes, sitting with rejection still sucks. There are mornings I still feel hollow. But now, I meet that hollow with curiosity: *What is it saying? What is it inviting?*

CHAPTER 7

A friend messaged me after a major corporate presentation. She said my calmness changed how her presentation landed. Her message: "I want to lead like that—without forcing respect, without hustling for validation. You taught me something I didn't know I needed."

If my presence modeled something possible for another person—something they could absorb—it meant I was living proof: you don't have to push to create impact.

So, why does softness create direction? Because it anchors in the root chakra of intuition. It comes from strength aligned with humility. It's a signature frequency that invites instead of commands.

In relational alchemy, I noticed push patterns—trying to earn love or acceptance. The antidote: presence energy. Show up, breathe, speak calmly. Let the other person recalibrate to your gifted space—not through manipulation, but through resonance. They felt heard. They leaned in.

I practiced small disruptions to my usual patterns. At a family dinner, I noticed my default "over-function" kicking in—cleaning plates, reminding people of logistics. My chest tightened again. I paused. I handed the napkins instead of piling them. I said: "Give me five minutes to just sit." They hesitated briefly, then smiled. The evening felt lighter. No one thought I was weak. They thought I was present.

In a coaching session, instead of jumping with strategy tips, I told my client: *"I want to hear how this feels to you."* Silence followed. Words emerged. Connection deepened. Clarity showed up. She felt seen—because I had *seen* her, by seeing myself.

One afternoon, I sat in traffic and felt my mind spinning, catching up on mistakes, next steps, contingency plans. I slowly tuned into the hum of the engine, the vibration in the steering wheel, the sound of my breath. For the first time, I didn't distract myself with a podcast. I just *was*. I felt layers loosen. I realized I could travel anywhere emotionally—and still land in presence. This was freedom.

Presence also means boundaries. Softness doesn't mean availability. I learned to say no to disruptions after dinner, no to overcommitting, no to text chains that siphoned my calm. Saying no from presence didn't feel weak—it felt sovereign.

The most subtle shift of all: I no longer ask permission. When I take up space—on camera, in conversation, in negotiations—I own my presence. Meeting rooms breathe differently. My voice shapes the tone, not from volume, but from grounded resonance.

In one pivotal negotiation, I used presence as my strategy. When questions arose, I paused, shifted my weight between feet, opened my hands—allowing space. The energy shifted from defense to collaboration. We reached an agreement that held respect, commitment, and warmth for both parties.

CHAPTER 7

That day I understood: presence is power. Quiet power. Power that builds bridges, not walls.

A few months later, I looked back on the crater of that email, the place of collapse. Now I understand: that collapse was blessing. It cracked me open. It removed the railings I didn't see I'd erected. And in the collapse, my pelvis softened, my spine found ease, my nervous system recalibrated from tension to alignment.

Presence gave me a new operating system. I still care about success, but I no longer chase my worth. I cultivate calm. I hold boundaries. I rise by presence, not by proving.

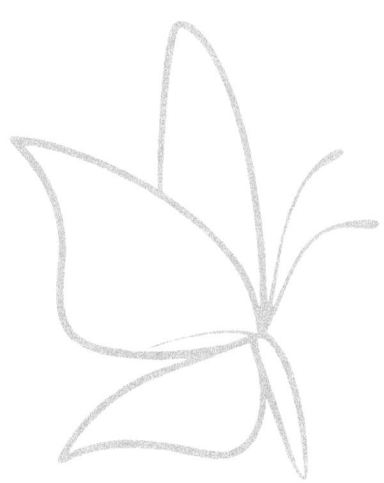

INVISIBLE PAIN, UNSTOPPABLE POWER

🌿 CORE PRACTICE TO ANCHOR PRESENCE & POWER

1. **Morning Stillness (5 min):**
   Sit upright, hands open. Label thoughts "story." Return to breath.

2. **Sensory Scanning (1 min):**
   Check jaw, shoulders, belly. Breathe into tension. Release.

3. **Presence Pledge (30 sec):**
   Whisper to yourself: *"I show up by being, not seeking."*

4. **Evening Reflection (3–5 min):**
   Write one place you practiced presence. How did it affect your interactions?

5. **Boundary Whisper:**
   Each day, identify a place to speak or rest from presence instead of performance.

When I bring presence into my leadership, I lead differently. When I bring it into my relationships, I connect differently. When I bring it into my own body, I heal differently.

Power does not diminish with softness—it amplifies with presence. This is how Invisible Pain became Unstoppable Power. This is how rejection became my rebirth.

CHAPTER 7

Your challenge isn't performance—it's presence. You are invited to descend into quiet. To soften your edges. To let your nervous system lead you back to your center. The world won't always change, but *you will*. And that is enough to change everything.

REFLECTIVE PROMPTS, VISUALS & BLANK PAGES

Add your reflection below:

Page ____:

Page ____:

Page ____:

Page ____:

Page ____:

NOTES

CHAPTER 8
EMBODIED SELF-TRUST: LISTENING TO YOUR INNER COMPASS

*"In every walk with nature,
one receives far more than he seeks."*
— JOHN MUIR

I grew up in a household where disagreements erupted like storms. Voices would rise to a pitch, eyes glazed with hurt and blame. We didn't just argue—we performed operatic battles of wills, where each person had to "win." Over time, I absorbed a script: to survive, you had to shout, escalate, or retreat into silence.

Years later, as I began healing my chronic pain and endometriosis, I realized something fundamental: disagreements don't have to implode into chaos. You can disagree without it being a shouting match. You can bear two perspectives and still love someone. Emotional honesty doesn't mean conflict; it means connection.

But if you never learn this, emotions wait. They simmer. They fester. They either burst into anger—or calcify into resentment and bitterness that poison relationships from within. I learned the hard way.

I carried bottled feelings for years—small everyday hurts, niggling frustration, disappointment in not being heard. Then came the breaking point: a close friend mentioned something that triggered one of those buried emotions, and suddenly I was screaming, words spilling out like toxic confessions. Afterwards, guilt settled in: *Why didn't I say this when it mattered? Why was I so quiet?*

My therapist offered a phrase that changed everything: *It can either become your excuse... or your reason.* That funerary, quiet grief of unspoken pain—was it a story of victimhood or a stepping-stone to self-mastery? I chose the latter. I decided I wanted to be a master of my destiny, not a victim of my history.

I began to unpack each emotional detonation: What was the feeling? Anger? Fear? Shame? Had it been triggered by something similar in my past? Most importantly, I started saying the words out loud in safe spaces: "I feel X when Y." No blame. Just owning my experience.

As I did this, I discovered something else: having grace under pressure, softness under stress, was not weakness—it was radical strength. I sat in business meetings and when tension rose, I didn't lean in with aggression. Instead, I breathed, I listened, I allowed silence to speak. Silence doesn't equate to emptiness—it can be full, connective, sovereign. That is power.

The power of listening—and belief in your own worthiness to feel. This is embodied self-trust—trusting your inner compass, allowing your intuition and sensations to become your guides.

This echoes the Heroine's Journey: after mastering the masculine realm of achievements and logic, you descend into the depths—embodiment, soul, intuition—and emerge with integration:

BUT HOW DO YOU CULTIVATE SELF-TRUST?

1. **Name the Emotion.**
   Catch it in your body: "Tongue tight? Heart pounding?" Stop and name it: *"That's anxiety."* Acknowledge it: *"I feel unseen."* Naming softens the narrative, separates you from the reactivity.

2. **Meet it with Kindness.**
   Instead of punishing: *"I shouldn't feel like this,"* pause and affirm: *"It's okay to feel this."* Kindness invites conversation; judgment shuts it down.

3. **Speak Before It Becomes a Storm.**

   "I feel hurt when you dismissed my idea." Hard as it is, speaking in the moment prevents internal seeding of resentment. Communication is not confrontation—it's mutual gravity.

4. **Pause Into Presence.**

   Learn to tolerate ambiguity. Silence doesn't need to be filled. In fact, in moments of discord, a calm pause can show more presence, control, and strength than words ever could.

5. **Lean Into Sensual Awareness.**

   Not sexual, but multi-sensory. Tune in: *"I feel tension in my shoulders, a cool breeze on my skin, the sunlight on my cheek."* This places you in your body—and in your power.

6. **Honor Thresholds.**

   Recognize your limits—not as weaknesses, but as wisdom. "I need five minutes before responding," or "I'm too tired to dig into this now—can we revisit tomorrow?" Boundaries are basic acts of self-trust.

These practices create the architecture of internal guidance: you start to feel safe with yourself. You begin to discover that your intuition is not whim—it's clarity in your cell memory. It's a thermostat, not a thermostat adjusting to the room—it is the room.

Through this, you stop living reactive lives. You stop replaying the old story from your upbringing. Instead, you claim sovereignty over how you feel—and how you respond.

One day, in a coaching session, I watched my client's whole posture shift as she named an emotion rather than burying it. She looked at me and said, *"This feels like lightness."* That's embodiment. That's self-trust resonating through your cells.

Another day, in a high-stakes negotiation, I didn't feel the need to prove everything. I just sat calmly, absorbing feedback, offering my truth when asked. And the deal emerged—not from pressure, but from mutual respect.

Opponents don't want to argue—you can disagree and still hold people alive in your heart. That's embodied integrity.

If you want to feel less reactive, less chaotic, more aligned—to trust yourself in pressure, to communicate calmly, to stand soft when everything wants hardness—then you need this: the cultivation of embodied self-trust.

EXERCISE: LISTENING TO YOUR INNER COMPASS

Part A – Body Awareness (5 minutes)
Close your eyes. Slowly scan from head to toe. Notice tension, warmth, coolness, vibration. Breathe into any area with tension. Say: *"I feel ___ in my body."*

Part B – Naming & Kindness
Recall a minor conflict from today (even with yourself). Without judgment, name the emotion: *"I felt hurt."* Then say: *"It's okay to feel hurt."*

Part C – Journal Prompt
Write one sentence: *"In moments of tension, I want to remember that listening within is my greatest strength."*

Part D – Micro-Boundary Statement
Next time you sense rising tension (inner or outer), say: *"Pause—I need a moment."* No drama. Just a statement of self-trust.

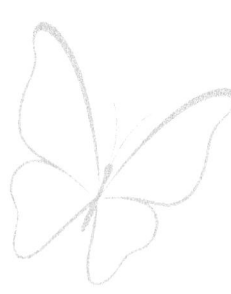

CHAPTER 8

YOUR INVITATION:

Through this practice, you build a body-deep faith in your inner witness. You prove to yourself again and again: I can show up—without performance. I can feel—without implosion. I can hold myself—and therefore hold others.

Let Chapter 7 be your portal into self-trust. Not stories, not affirmations, but embodied truth. You feel, you speak, you rest when needed. You don't collapse, but you don't fight either. You become *the calm, the container, the clarity.*

And when you trust yourself—truly, deeply—you'll never be lost again.

CALL TO ACTION: THE INNER COMPASS ACTIVATION

Today, you've learned how to hold yourself in emotional tension with grace—not letting your history define you. Now it's time to go deeper.

I challenge you: In the next week, **choose one real-life disagreement or stress moment**—it could be at work, in a relationship, or with yourself. **Instead of reacting, follow the Inner Compass Activation sequence below**, and **journal your experience** afterward.

INNER COMPASS ACTIVATION SEQUENCE

1. **Drop Physical Armor (1 minute)**

   Find a quiet spot. Stand or sit tall. Do a gentle **Chair Yoga Side Stretch** or **Boat Pose** (navasana) to open your core and relieve tension—physically **release stiffness, and lower your cortisol response** (victorianhan.com, stevie-wright.com, vogue.com). This prepares your body to feel, not armor up.

2. **Sensory Grounding (30 seconds)**

   Engage your senses: **see, hear, touch, smell, taste**—use the 5-4-3-2-1 method to bring your body into the here and now.

3. **Feel & Name (1 minute)**

   Notice emotional waves—anger, hurt, frustration. Place your hand on your heart and name: "**This is** _____." Research says naming emotion activates self-healing pathways and strengthens neural integration.

4. **Pause & Embodied Breath (30 seconds)**

   Breathe slowly into your belly for 10 cycles. Let shoulders and jaw relax. At the exhale, mentally whisper: *"I stay clear, I stay present."*

5. **Speak from Presence**

   Return embodying this grounded self. With calm clarity, express: "**When** _____ **happens, I feel** _____. **I need** _____." No escalation, no surrender—just sovereignty.

6. **Celebrate the Shift**

   Observe what changed: Did silence invite more composure? Did your words land clearer? Did you feel strength in softness?

JOURNAL INTEGRATION

Right after:

1. Describe what happened.

---

2. Rate your nervous system before (1–10) and after the process.

---

3. What surprised you about staying embodied and speaking from presence?

---

4. What shift did you sense—in yourself or from others?

CHAPTER 8

THE UNIQUE POWER OF THIS PRACTICE

This isn't another mindfulness exercise. It's a **somatic initiation**—blending proven postural release (Boat Pose/Chair Yoga) with sensory grounding and emotional naming. It anchors your **inner compass** in body + mind alignment—so when your history rises, **you no longer default to old stories.** You lead from presence.

YOUR PURPOSE

By doing this with even one conflict this week, you'll begin to **prove to yourself, cell by cell**, that you can:

- Feel hard feelings without fracturing
- Speak your truth without slipping into old dramas
- Be centered, not silenced; clear, not reactive

That's embodied self-trust—and once rooted, it unlocks your ability to navigate *any* pressure moment with grounded sovereignty.

Let this exercise be your initiation into a new way of living: **from your axis, not your armor.** Do it consciously. Do it fully. And write down what shifts.

Because once you **activate your inner compass**, you'll never be lost—or led—again.

CHAPTER 9

THE TRUTH BENEATH THE PAIN: RECLAIMING POWER THROUGH THE FEMININE

"One you make a decision, the universe conspires to make it happen."
— RALPH WALDO EMERSON

I used to think I was broken.

I didn't say that out loud, of course. I buried it deep—under layers of performance, perfectionism, and people-pleasing. I wore confidence like a mask. I mastered my resume, sharpened my words, and looked the part. But underneath it all, my body was at war with me—and I was at war with myself.

Body dysmorphia. Endometriosis. Chronic pain.

You don't "wake up" one day with these things. They creep in silently, gradually, until they become a language your body speaks fluently—and the world refuses to understand.

But this is not a story of suffering. This is a story of **alchemy**.

And if you've been hiding your pain behind your power—or worse, pretending you're fine when you're falling apart—this is for you.

CHAPTER 9

THE PAIN THAT DOESN'T BLEED

Endometriosis isn't just painful—it's invisible. That's what makes it so maddening.

You learn to normalize agony. You show up at work while your body feels like it's tearing itself apart. You fake smiles on dates while you're swallowing nausea and shame. You hide hot water bottles under your desk and pop Advil like it's candy just to make it through lunch.

I was told it was "just period pain." That it was in my head. That I was being dramatic.

So I believed them. And then I believed something far worse: I thought maybe I wasn't strong enough.

That lie will eat you alive. And for years, it almost did.

Until I decided that if the pain wasn't going anywhere, I wasn't going to waste another second being ashamed of it.

I was going to **alchemize** it.

That was the moment I stepped into a power I didn't know I had.

REWRITING THE NARRATIVE

Healing doesn't begin with answers. It begins with permission.

I gave myself permission to stop fighting my body and start listening to it.
I gave myself permission to cry, to scream, to cancel, to say no.
I gave myself permission to want more.

Most importantly, I gave myself permission to be both: strong and soft, driven and delicate, in control and in surrender.

This wasn't about pretending everything was okay. It was about understanding that my value wasn't tied to how well I could perform while silently suffering.

It was time to stop hiding.

You don't need to "prove" your power.
You already **are** it.

CHAPTER 9

THE FEMININE POWER WE FORGOT

We live in a world that praises masculine achievement. Hustle. Push. Conquer. Control.

And listen—I love building empires and breaking glass ceilings as much as the next woman. But there's a quiet superpower we've been conditioned to suppress: the **feminine**.

Feminine energy is not weakness. It is not passive. It is magnetic. Receptive. Creative. Intuitive. Healing.

Feminine power does not scream for attention—it **attracts** with intention.

And when you learn how to embody it, not only do you stop chasing—you start receiving.

That was one of the most life-changing mindset shifts of my journey: *Reception is a strength.*

THE ALCHEMY OF PAIN

Alchemy is not magic. It's transformation.

In ancient times, alchemists tried to turn lead into gold. But real alchemy?
It happens in the heart.

When I finally saw my pain not as a curse but as a crucible, everything changed.
My symptoms became my teachers.
My scars became maps.
My suffering became sacred.

Pain is the fire. Power is the gold.

There's a kind of strength that can't be bought—only earned.
It's the kind that says:
I went through the fire, and I came out with light.

When you embrace your pain as part of your path—not your identity—you shift from victim to visionary.

BENEFITS AND DRAWBACKS OF THE EVENT

Let me be transparent.

The drawbacks:

- I lost time. Time in bed. Time crying. Time others used to live freely.
- I lost trust. In my body. In practitioners. In relationships that couldn't hold space for me.
- I lost illusions—naïve ideas that the body should never break.

But the benefits?

- I gained empathy so deep it makes strangers feel like family.
- I gained resilience that can't be taught in schools.
- I gained purpose—a sacred mission. A voice rooted in truth.

And here's the wildest part:

I wouldn't trade it.

COMPANION PRACTICE: TRUTH TRANSMUTATION

This isn't just journaling. It's a ceremony.

A sacred rewriting of your own nervous system. An energetic recalibration through language. It's how I alchemized pain on the page.

STEP 1: THE TRIGGER

Write down one raw sentence. The thing you're afraid to say.

"I feel invisible."
"I feel unworthy."
"I'm tired of pretending I'm okay."

STEP 2: THE TRUTH

Now write what your **higher self** would say.

"My worth isn't defined by validation."
"I am seen by the divine."
"My pain matters."

STEP 3: THE TRANSMUTATION

Turn your trigger + truth into a paragraph that turns pain into power.

"Even when I feel invisible, I radiate presence. I am not here to be small. I am here to light rooms, not beg to be noticed."

Write it in your voice. Say it like you mean it. Make it yours.

STEP 4: EMBODY IT

Place your hand on your heart, womb, or wherever you carry emotion. Speak the paragraph out loud.
Let the words land in your cells.

Say it again.
And again.

Let your body believe you.

STEP 5: ANCHOR AND REPEAT

Do this **daily** for 21 days.

- Add soft music.
- Light a candle.
- Use breathwork: inhale peace, exhale pain.
- Look into a mirror and say it to yourself.

You are not journaling.
You are **reprogramming your frequency**.
You are writing as medicine.
You are returning to yourself.

CHAPTER 9

QUANTUM TRUTH: ENERGY, EMOTION, AND ALCHEMY

Everything is energy.

Every thought. Every word. Every tear. Every diagnosis.

Pain holds frequency. So does love.

Once I stopped viewing pain as punishment and began viewing it as **information**, I stopped resisting it. I started reading it. Responding to it. Learning from it.

Energy can't be destroyed. But it can be **transformed**.

You don't have to recycle pain anymore.
You can rise through it.

CALL TO ACTION: THE SHIFT STARTS NOW

If this chapter stirred something in you, it's not by accident.

You are ready.

Ready to stop shrinking.
Ready to stop chasing
Ready to stop apologizing.
Ready to **remember who the f*ck you are.**

So here's your soul invitation:

1. **Write your permission slip.**
   You don't need the world's blessing—just your own.

2. **Get radically honest.**
   Truth is your medicine.

3. **Feel it to free it.**
   Let the emotions pass through, not stay stuck.

4. **Speak your story.**
   Your voice heals.

5. **Receive.**
   You are magnetic when you stop chasing.

6. **Practice your rituals.**
   Light candles. Breathe. Move. Speak.

7. **Use the Truth Transmutation practice**
   as often as needed.

8. **Trust the alchemy.**
   You are not lost. You are becoming.

You were never broken.
You were becoming.

Your pain was never the end.
It was the **initiation**.

And now, it's time to rise.

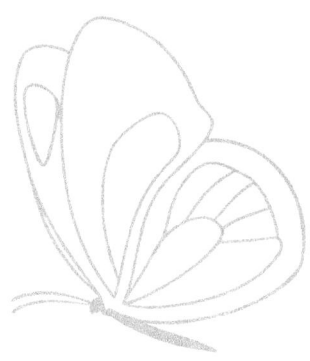

NOTES

NOTES

CHAPTER 10
THE SCIENCE OF SELF ADVOCACY

"At the center of your being you have the answer, you know who you are and you know what you want."
— Lao Tzu

There comes a moment in everyone's life—particularly those who have suffered in silence for years—when you realize no one is coming to rescue you. No white horse. No perfect doctor. No final diagnosis that suddenly makes it all make sense. That moment, while terrifying, is also the most liberating. Because it's in that moment that you realize: **I must become my own advocate.**

Let us talk about that shift—from disempowered to powerful, from voiceless to vocal, from invisible to undeniable. This is

The Science of Self-Advocacy, and it's not just a mindset. It's a skill, a practice, a discipline, and ultimately, a revolution.

Let's get something clear from the beginning: self-advocacy is not about being loud. It's about being clear. It's not about confrontation for the sake of drama; it's about **conscious confrontation** when your well-being is on the line. In fact, self-advocacy begins long before you utter a single word. It starts with **self-permission**: to matter, to speak, to ask, to challenge, and to redirect the energy around you.

It begins the moment you choose to shift your mindset from victim to witness. From: "Why is this happening to me?" to: "This is happening. What do I choose to do with it?"

RECLAIMING THE POWER OF PERCEPTION

One of the most important pivots on the path to self-advocacy is reclaiming **how we perceive our circumstances**. The old programming says: life is hard, you get what you get, be grateful for crumbs, and don't rock the boat.

But what if the boat was never yours to begin with?

Self-advocacy demands you stop tolerating the intolerable. Not through rage (although sometimes anger is justified), but through clarity. When we choose to shift our perception from *powerless participant* to *conscious creator*, everything changes.

Pain isn't personal. It's just a signal.

It doesn't mean you're broken. It means you're receiving information. And once you understand that, you stop gaslighting yourself. You start validating your own experience. That's the gateway to power.

CHOOSING YOUR NARRATIVE

One of the most critical aspects of self-advocacy is **narrative control**. We all have stories we tell ourselves:

- "I'm not strong enough."
- "No one believes me."
- "I'm always too much or not enough."

These stories become internal laws. But guess what? **You're the legislator.** You can repeal the ones that don't serve you.

As I have shared before, I was anemic and terrified, with IVs in both arms and fear coursing through me, I had a choice: sink into my self-pity or reframe her circumstances. I chose laughter. I chose connection. I chose the mindset of *survivor*, not *victim*.

That shift changed my chemistry. It altered the tone of the entire experience. And it birthed a new relationship with my own strength.

ACCOUNTABILITY: THE HARDEST PILL TO SWALLOW

Self-advocacy asks something radical of us: **accountability**. And this is where most people opt out. Because the moment you recognize that you are responsible for your responses, you can no longer hide behind blame.

It's easier to say, "the system is broken," than to say, "how am I complicit in my own silencing?"

But here's the beauty: **once you take responsibility, you reclaim your freedom.** You get to write new scripts. You get to pause, pivot, and rise.

This isn't about toxic positivity. It's about sovereign self-responsibility.

TOOLS OF SELF-ADVOCACY

1. RADICAL SELF-AWARENESS

Start with emotional literacy. Where in your body do you feel tension? What patterns do you repeat when stressed? Whose voice are you hearing when you doubt yourself?

Awareness is 80% of the work. Because what you're aware of, you can change. What you're unaware of, controls you.

2. LANGUAGE UPGRADE

Stop diminishing yourself:

- Replace "I'm sorry, but..." with "Thank you for your patience."
- Replace "I think..." with "I believe..."
- Replace "If it's not too much trouble..." with "This is what I need."

Language is your leadership.
Words cast spells. Speak powerfully.

3. THE EMOTIONAL RESET

Learn to regulate. Breathwork. Journaling. Walking in nature. These aren't luxuries—they're lifelines. When your nervous system is calm, your boundaries are clear.

You cannot advocate for yourself from a dysregulated state. Calm is your superpower.

4. SAY NO, WITHOUT THE STORY

You don't need a paragraph to justify your no. "No" is a complete sentence. So is "I'm not available for that." Or "That doesn't work for me."

Self-advocacy requires that you disappoint others *before* you betray yourself.

5. REWRITE THE IDENTITY

I shared how I once thought I had a low pain threshold—until doctors confirmed that I had been living with one of the most painful conditions on the planet. I didn't have a low tolerance. I had a **high threshold for survival.**

That is not weakness. That is warriorhood.

Self-advocacy often begins the moment you realize: *I am stronger than I gave myself credit for.*

BREAKING THROUGH INTERNAL BARRIERS

What holds most people back from advocating for themselves? Shame. Fear. The belief that they're not worth it.

But consider this: **Would you talk to your 3-year-old self the way you talk to yourself now?** Would you let someone treat her the way you allow others to treat you?

Self-advocacy is remembering that **you are still that child**. Still worthy. Still whole. Still sacred.

Place a photo of yourself as a child where you can see it. Make her your standard.

FROM PAIN CYCLE TO POWER CYCLE

For years, I felt trapped in a cycle of suffering—self-pity, helplessness, and a body that seemed to betray me at every turn. What I didn't realize then was that my nervous system had been programmed to rehearse pain, replaying trauma long after the wound had passed. I described centralized pain syndrome—where trauma in one part of the body leads to ongoing, amplified pain. This isn't imagined. It's neurological. But the blessing is this: pain can be transmuted into your greatest gifts. Just as pain can become programmed, so can peace.

We can train ourselves to reframe. To breathe through triggers. To insert space between stimulus and response. To elevate our energy in the middle of discomfort. Every choice you make is a vote for your future. Every breath, a signal to your nervous system: you are safe, you are strong, you are capable of healing. And from this shift, the Pain Cycle to Power Cycle was born.

I am safe.
I am whole.
I am healing.

DAILY ADVOCACY PRACTICE

1. MORNING MANTRA:

- I am my own greatest advocate.
- I trust my body.
- I speak my truth clearly and with love.

2. MIRROR AFFIRMATIONS:

- "My pain is real."
- "This too shall pass."
- "I am not broken. I am a miracle in motion."

3. 5-MINUTE JOURNALING PROMPT:

- Where am I abandoning myself?
- What does my body need today?
- What boundary needs reinforcing?

4. EMBODIMENT PRACTICE:

- Movement: stretch, dance, walk.
- Breath: 4-7-8 breathing cycle (inhale 4, hold 7, exhale 8)
- Stillness: 2 minutes in silence, hand on heart.

Repeat for 21 days and track your transformation.

CHAPTER 10

QUOTES FOR ANCHORING YOUR POWER

"Once you make a decision, the universe conspires to make it happen."
—RALPH WALDO EMERSON

"Shift happens."
—UNKNOWN

"The most important decision you will ever make is to be in a good mood."
—VOLTAIRE

"I am whole, alive, and well."
—MLK, INSPIRED

"Enjoy your holiday on Earth."
—EARL NIGHTINGALE

"The first wealth is health."
—RALPH WALDO EMERSON

FINAL THOUGHTS

Self-advocacy is not a one-time act. It's a daily devotion to truth. A radical reclamation of worth. It is the practice of remembering that your voice is sacred. Your pain is valid. Your story is power.

No one will speak for you the way *you* can. No one will fight for your life the way *you* must. But here's the good news: you're not alone. Every time you rise, you rise for those who are still finding their voice.

You rise for your past self. You rise for the future. You rise for truth.

And that, dear reader, is how invisible pain becomes unstoppable power. Transmute the energy, change your perception as perception is your reality!

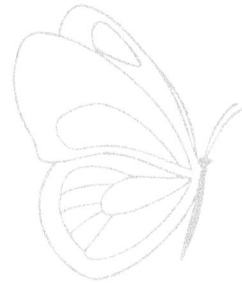

NOTES

NOTES

NOTES

CHAPTER 11
FAITH, PURPOSE & THE SPIRITUAL PATH TO HEALING

"Mastering yourself is true power."
—Lao Tzu

Navigating the healthcare system can often feel cold and clinical — not because every doctor lacks compassion, but because the system itself can unintentionally strip away the human element. Yet, in the midst of that sterility, there are moments of deep humanity. One patient recalled a surgeon — a man who, informed by his wife's experiences, took the time to acknowledge the pain she was in. He didn't just operate; he empathized. And that, sometimes, is the most healing medicine of all: to be seen, heard, and understood.

While there are many remarkable physicians doing their best within a rigid system, women's pain is still too often misunderstood or dismissed. Whether it's limited pain relief after major procedures or assumptions that downplay our experience, the gap is real. But so is the growing movement to shift this narrative.

This book is part of that movement.

To change the world outside us, we first have to strengthen what's within us. And that begins with faith.

FAITH AS FOUNDATION

Faith has been an anchor in my life — not the kind tied to a specific religion, but a deep trust in something greater. I was raised in the Soviet Union during a time when religion was banned. There were no churches. I was raised atheist, disconnected from traditional spirituality. It wasn't until after the fall of the Soviet regime that I started going to church with my grandfather. Even then, it didn't feel like home. I didn't understand it.

But over time, patterns emerged in my life. Patterns that I could not ignore. Wishes I didn't get — and thank God I didn't — because in hindsight, what I thought I wanted would've hurt me. And that's when I started to believe. Not in dogma, but in design. I saw the intelligent organization of nature, the synchronicities, the quiet wisdom. And I started to surrender — to trust that everything happens for a reason.

CHAPTER 11

I wouldn't erase a single piece of my journey, no matter how painful. Endometriosis. Body dysmorphia. Trauma. I wouldn't wish those experiences on anyone, but I also wouldn't trade them — because they made me who I am.

FAITH + ACTION = MANIFESTATION

Faith, to me, is not passive. It's not about sitting back and waiting for the universe to show up like Amazon Prime. It's about co-creating. You have to do your part. You have to move your feet, take the steps. Want to meet the love of your life? Then leave your house. Take inspired action. Faith without works is fantasy.

There's a quote that's always stuck with me: *"Once you make a decision, the universe conspires to make it happen."* But you have to decide. You have to become the person who aligns with the life you want. That means healing. That means showing up. That means releasing what doesn't serve you so you can hold space for what does.

THE FEAR THAT BLOCKS US

So what keeps us from trusting the journey? Fear. Plain and simple. Fear of failure. Fear that it won't work out. Fear that we're not enough.

But fear is a liar. It's also a teacher. And it's usually loudest right before a breakthrough. The secret? Start anyway. Mark Twain said, *"The secret of getting ahead is getting started."* Most people never do. They spend their energy imagining all the ways they could fail, instead of visualizing what it would feel like to win.

When you trust that the universe has your back, the fear starts to lose its grip. Life becomes less about control and more about flow.

WHEN THE UNIVERSE SPEAKS

I've had moments — real, visceral moments — when I felt the universe speak to me. One in particular stands out.

As I have shared before, during the pandemic, I created a small garden sanctuary. I went to a nursery and felt compelled to pick up a milkweed plant — the food source for monarch butterflies. I didn't know why. It didn't match the rest of my plants. But I bought it.

Days later, I found tiny caterpillars eating the leaves. Monarch butterfly larvae. I ended up raising 13 butterflies. I watched them form cocoons. I watched them hatch. One had a broken wing and couldn't fly, so we kept him as a pet for a month.

And all the while, I was going through my own transformation — confronting decades of self-image issues, reclaiming my worth, choosing to love myself. Those butterflies were more than nature. They were messengers. Symbols of the metamorphosis happening within me. This miracle of nature stayed with me to this day, I grow a milkweed garden every year to never forget magic of those butterflies transformation and what it feels like to have them emerge and, crawl right onto your hand...

It was the universe saying: *You're ready. Stop hiding. Shine.*

STRENGTHENING INTUITION

If you want to hear the universe, you need to turn down the volume of the world. During lockdown, I finally had the quiet I needed to hear my inner voice. For years, it had been drowned out by noise — social media, news, expectations, opinions. But in that stillness, I found clarity. THIS is where my healing journey began- in lockdown I found the stillness to begin my own transformation, that's when I planted my garden that became a sanctuary for endangered monarch butterflies.

We were not designed to absorb as much external input as we do today. Constant stimulation kills intuition. Silence revives it. Solitude sharpens it. That's why practices like journaling, nature walks, and digital detoxes are more than self-care — they're spiritual hygiene.

GRATITUDE: THE FREQUENCY OF RECEIVING

Gratitude is more than a virtue. It's a vibration. When you are truly grateful, you align with abundance. You match the energy of receiving.

I remember listening to Gregg Braden speak about manifesting rain. He didn't *ask* for rain. He imagined himself *feeling grateful* for the rain that already was. That's how powerful gratitude is.

During my personal transformation, I began reconnecting with my inner child — the one who loved nature, horseback riding, cookies. That child was naturally joyful. Naturally grateful. And I began to see: gratitude isn't something you acquire. It's something you remember.

LIVING ON PURPOSE

Do I believe we all have a purpose? Yes. Without question. Can I prove it? No. But I feel it. And when you're aligned with your purpose, you'll know. You'll feel it in your body. There's a peace that comes, a calm. Things begin to flow. You stop chasing. You start allowing.

I left the corporate world because it made me sick — literally. My body revolted. Migraines. Nausea. Exhaustion. Secrets I couldn't keep. Ethics I couldn't swallow. I knew it wasn't my path.

CHAPTER 11

Purpose feels like coming home to yourself. It feels like the freedom to breathe fully. It feels like joy — not the fleeting kind, but the rooted, soul-satisfying kind.

I believe we're not just here to survive. We're here to feel fulfilled. And fulfillment comes when we stop chasing someone else's definition of success and start living our own.

So take the step. Do the thing. Say the prayer. Plant the seed. The universe is listening.

And if you're still unsure?

Look for the butterflies.

REFLECTION & ACTION EXERCISE: ACTIVATE YOUR FAITH, FUEL YOUR FLOW

1. Name three things you're grateful for today:
Write them out with as much feeling as possible. Gratitude anchors you in the present and activates abundance.

2. Notice the abundance in your life:
Write 10 examples of abundance around you right now — it could be time, love, nature, food, friendship, energy, or even the breath in your lungs.

3. Write your top three desires and goals for today:
Be specific. Let your soul guide your list. These can be big or small. What do you most want to create, experience, or move forward?

4. Identify your top three traits you love about yourself:
Self-love is magnetic. Celebrate the qualities that make you unique and powerful.

5. Now go take action — with grace, love, and courage.
One step. One conversation. One aligned move. You don't have to see the whole staircase — just take the next step.

You got this.

NOTES

NOTES

CHAPTER 11

INTEGRATION EXERCISE: ALIGNING WITH FAITH, PURPOSE & GRATITUDE

Transformation isn't just something we talk about — it's something we embody. Let's take the insights from this chapter and turn them into **tangible, soulful action**.

1. NAME THREE THINGS YOU'RE GRATEFUL FOR

Gratitude is the frequency of miracles. Pause. Breathe. And anchor into appreciation.

- _____
- _____
- _____
- _____
- _____
- _____
- _____

2. NOTICE THE ABUNDANCE AROUND YOU

Look around.
You're already surrounded by more than you realize.

Write down **ten signs of abundance** in your life right now — they could be physical, emotional, spiritual, or even symbolic.

1. _____

2. _____

3. _____

4. _____

5. _____

6. _____

7. _____

8. _____

9. _____

10. _____

3. WRITE YOUR TOP THREE DESIRES OR GOALS FOR TODAY

Focus on what you *want* — not what you fear. Your intention shapes your reality.

What three things do you want to move toward **today**, even if it's one small step?

- _____
  _____
  _____

- _____
  _____
  _____

- _____
  _____
  _____

4. OWN YOUR GREATNESS:
PICK 3 TRAITS YOU LOVE ABOUT YOURSELF

You are already enough. You've got gifts the world needs. Name three traits you deeply love and admire about YOU.

- _____

  _____

  _____

- _____

  _____

  _____

- _____

  _____

  _____

5. NOW TAKE ACTION — WITH GRACE, LOVE, AND COURAGE

The universe responds to movement. Even one aligned action can change your trajectory.

Choose one of your desires above, and commit to **one action** you will take today.

Then say this out loud (yes, really!):

"I am divinely guided.
I take bold, loving action in alignment with my purpose.
I trust the process.
I trust myself.
Let's go!"

You've got this.
The next chapter of your life starts now.

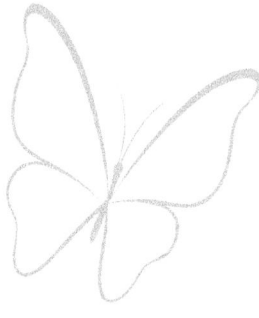

CHAPTER 12

LIVING UNSTOPPABLE – INTEGRATING POWER ACROSS EVERY ROLE

"When I let go of what I am, I become what I might be."
—Lao Tzu

In a world that demands constant evolution, true power is not found in brute strength or dominance — but in fluidity, grace, boundaries, and unwavering presence. Living an unstoppable life means harnessing every part of who you are — the leader, the mother, the partner, the creator, and the healer — and learning to navigate those roles with intention and self-awareness.

For so long, the narrative around success has been linear: achieve, conquer, repeat. But what if unstoppable power isn't about conquering at all? What if it's about alignment? About coming home to yourself in every room you enter, every decision you make, every boundary you hold?

This chapter is about how to fully embody your unstoppable self — not just at work or on stage, but in the kitchen, in your quiet moments, in love, in loss, and in transition. This is the integration.

LEADERSHIP REDEFINED

Leadership isn't a title. It's not a nameplate on a desk or the loudest voice in the room. Leadership is energy. It's how you hold yourself, how you listen, how you lift others.

Unstoppable leaders are not afraid of vulnerability. They know when to ask for help, when to pause, and when to roar. They lead by example, not by force.

Redefining leadership means:

- Leading with empathy, not ego
- Listening to understand, not to respond
- Making space for others to rise
- Knowing your values — and living by them
- Setting boundaries that protect your peace and purpose

When you integrate power across roles, your leadership becomes embodied. You lead your team, your children, your clients, and yourself from the same rooted energy.

MOTHERHOOD AND THE DIVINE FEMININE

Whether you are a mother, a nurturer, or a creator in any form, the energy of motherhood is powerful. It is the energy of origin — of creation, destruction, protection, and rebirth.

Unstoppable mothers know that caring for others begins with caring for themselves. They do not glorify burnout. They redefine what it means to be "strong."

You can be soft and strong.
You can cry and still be courageous.
You can ask for help and still be a warrior.

Integrating power in motherhood means:

- Releasing guilt as a measure of love
- Modeling boundaries to your children and community
- Choosing presence over perfection
- Honoring your needs without apology

Motherhood, when embodied with somatic awareness, becomes a daily spiritual practice. Every tantrum, every sleepless night, every lunch packed — becomes a sacred act of love when done with intention. I talked A LOT about how the idea of motherhood became transformational, I could no longer give birth to a child, it was hard to make peace with but I could give birth to other things, ideas, projects...

RELATIONSHIPS AS MIRRORS

Relationships are sacred mirrors. Whether romantic, familial, or platonic, the people we choose to be close to reflect our deepest wounds and our greatest gifts.

To live unstoppable in love means:

- Not shrinking for someone else's comfort
- Loving without losing yourself
- Choosing connection over codependence
- Speaking your truth — even when your voice shakes

Boundaries are a love language. They teach others how to treat us and remind us what we value.

Somatic cues to watch in relationship:

- Tight chest or shoulders when you're silencing yourself
- Gut tension when you're violating your own values
- Fatigue after spending time with certain people

Your body keeps the score. Trust it. Let it guide your relational decisions.

PUBLIC PRESENCE AND INNER ALIGNMENT

Being seen — truly seen — can be terrifying. Especially when you've spent years masking, adapting, pleasing.

Unstoppable public presence means:

- Letting your inner self match your outer voice
- Releasing the performance and stepping into authenticity
- Using your platform to serve, not to impress
- Showing up when it's hard, and resting when it's wise

You don't need to be everything to everyone. You need to be real. The world is starving for authenticity.

When your inner world is aligned, your public presence becomes magnetic.

MANAGING TRANSITIONS WITH GRACE

Every transformation is a death and a rebirth.

Divorce. Job change. Health crisis. Grief. New motherhood. Career shifts. These are not interruptions. These *are* the path.

Grace doesn't mean passive. It means present. It means trusting the season you're in, even when it's winter in your soul.

Somatic awareness during transitions can help you:

- Ground your nervous system
- Honor your body's natural rhythms
- Make space for integration

Somatic tools:

- Breathwork: 4 counts in, 7 hold, 8 out (activates parasympathetic nervous system)
- Walking meditations
- Grounding exercises (barefoot on grass, touching a tree, cold showers)

Your body is the portal through which transformation becomes embodied.

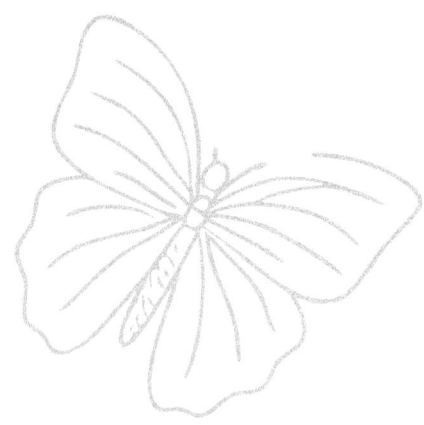

CHAPTER 12

REAL-LIFE CASE STUDIES: EVERYDAY UNSTOPPABLE POWER

CASE STUDY 1:
MARIA, SINGLE MOM & TECH LEADER

Maria, a single mom of two and a director in tech, redefined leadership by integrating her maternal instincts into her workplace. She started leading meetings with check-ins, implemented flexible hours for her team, and led with radical honesty. Her retention numbers improved by 30% and she was promoted to VP.

CASE STUDY 2:
DEVON, TRANS WOMAN & COMMUNITY ADVOCATE

Devon transitioned in her late 40s and used her visibility to empower others. She integrated her journey into her business speaking circuit, hosted workshops on identity and resilience, and created a mentorship program for LGBTQ+ youth. Her presence became her platform.

CASE STUDY 3:
NIA, BURNOUT SURVIVOR TURNED COACH

After collapsing from burnout, Nia took a year off, studied somatic therapy, and rebuilt her life from the inside out. She now runs a six-figure coaching practice focused on sustainable success for high-achieving women. Her mantra? "Slower is faster."

Unstoppable doesn't mean immune to pain. It means you don't stay down. You alchemize the breakdown into your next breakthrough.

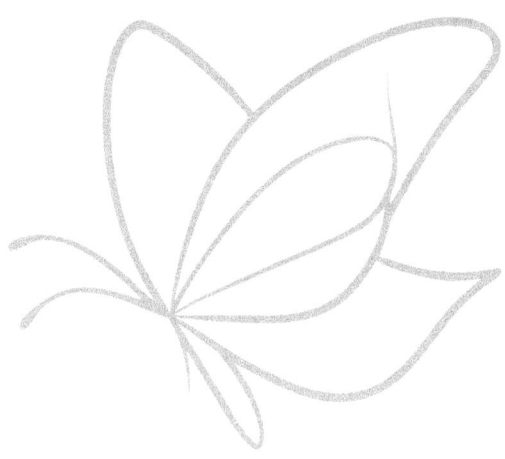

CHAPTER 12

BLUEPRINT FOR SUSTAINABLE TRANSFORMATION

Want to live unstoppable across every role? Here's your blueprint:

1. Self-Inquiry

- What roles am I playing out of obligation vs. alignment?
- Where do I shrink to fit?
- What does power feel like in my body?

2. Somatic Practice

- Start your day with breathwork or grounding
- Notice tension throughout the day — what's it saying?
- Close your day with body scans or intuitive movement

3. Boundary Setting

- Learn to say no with love, not guilt
- Create tech-free zones or hours
- Protect your non-negotiables (rest, food, pleasure)

4. Community and Support

- Surround yourself with those who reflect your highest self
- Hire a coach, therapist, or somatic practitioner
- Build a sisterhood or brotherhood of allies

5. **Purpose Reconnection**

- Journal weekly: What lit me up this week?
- Meditate on your future self and the life they live
- Celebrate micro-wins as evidence of momentum

Sustainable transformation is not about doing more. It's about doing what matters — deeply, consciously, unapologetically.

INTEGRATION EXERCISES

EXERCISE 1: GRATITUDE RECALIBRATION

- Write down **three things you're grateful for today.**
- Reflect on how they make you feel in your body.
- Ask: What abundance already surrounds me?

EXERCISE 2: POWER IN EVERY ROLE

- List **each of your key roles** (e.g., leader, mother, partner, friend, artist).
- Beside each, write **one way you show up in your power.**
- Identify **one area in each role where you want to improve.**

EXERCISE 3: SOMATIC BOUNDARY SETTING

- Take a moment to **sit quietly** and scan your body.
- Ask: Where am I holding tension?
- Visualize creating a **protective field** around yourself.
- Breathe into your belly and affirm:
  "I honor myself by choosing what aligns with my truth."

Living unstoppable is not about never falling. It's about rising with intention, every time. Across every role you hold — may you rise, rooted in truth, grace, and undeniable power.

RISING FROM THE ASHES

CELEBRATING THE ALCHEMY OF INVISIBLE PAIN

Pain has a peculiar way of shaping us—sharpening the dull edges of who we once were and forging a new self in the fires of suffering. When we speak of invisible pain—chronic illness, emotional trauma, unseen grief—we're not just speaking of symptoms. We're speaking of soul-forged transformation. And just like the phoenix myth told across cultures, we are meant to rise—burned, yes, but brilliant.

This chapter is both celebration and culmination. Whether you are a woman who has carried the weight of a silent battle or a man whose suffering never found space to speak, you are here now. Not just surviving—but awakening.

Let's dive deep into the full-spectrum radiance that comes when we turn pain into power and transformation into legacy.

PART I: FROM ASHES TO ALCHEMY — TRANSMUTING PAIN INTO PURPOSE

Alchemy, in its traditional sense, was about turning lead into gold. But true alchemy—spiritual alchemy—is about turning wounds into wisdom, trauma into truth, and scars into sacred symbols of growth.

Invisible pain often isolates us. It convinces us that we're broken, behind, or burdensome. But pain can be redefined. It can be seen as the threshold—a rite of passage into higher self-awareness, deeper compassion, and sacred resilience. Pain asks us to become more than what we thought we were. Not less. Never less.

Men and women alike suffer in silence. Men are often denied emotional literacy. Taught to "suck it up." Women, on the other hand, are often dismissed as "too emotional," "dramatic," or "hormonal." Both suffer in the margins. Both require radical permission to alchemize.

"What if your pain is not a punishment, but a portal?"

Pain invites us to slow down, to listen, to feel what we've avoided. It is the ultimate inner compass, if we allow it.

PART II: BLUEPRINT FOR RADIANCE — HOW WE HEAL AND STAY LIT

Healing is not a one-time event. It's a lifelong, layered reclamation. And the secret is this: your healing is not a detour from your purpose. It **is** the path.

1. Somatic Wisdom

The body keeps score, as Bessel van der Kolk reminded the world. Unprocessed trauma doesn't just vanish. It shows up in muscle tension, autoimmune responses, hormonal imbalance, and chronic fatigue. Whether you're male or female, the body becomes your sacred textbook. Learn its language.

- Practice breathwork to reset your nervous system.
- Dance. Shake. Move emotion through the body.
- Allow tears to flow—tears are chemical messengers that carry pain away.

2. Emotional Alchemy

Instead of numbing your anger, feel it. Beneath anger is often grief. Beneath grief is love. Emotional intelligence isn't about control—it's about fluency. Men, especially, are taught to bypass emotion. But it's emotional honesty that leads to emotional mastery.

3. Energetic Hygiene

Every interaction is an energy exchange. Boundaries are not walls—they are sacred contracts of self-respect. If something drains your energy, it doesn't belong in your life. Period.

Daily practices for energy:

- Grounding walks in nature
- Smudging with sage or palo santo
- Digital detox days
- Keeping your word to yourself

4. Legacy Activation

The healed version of you doesn't just feel better—you *build better*. You inspire, mentor, and create. Your healing creates ripple effects.

Your book, your story, your voice—they matter.

Every healed person becomes a lighthouse.

PART III: STORIES FROM THE FIRE — REAL VOICES, REAL POWER

Jared's Journey:
The Burnout Awakening (Male Perspective)

Jared, 43, was a C-suite executive who ignored the whispers of his body until they became screams. Panic attacks. Numbness in limbs. Emotional detachment from his children. It was only when he collapsed during a board meeting that he surrendered. He stepped away for six months, underwent somatic therapy, and began a journaling practice. He now coaches other high-performing men on how to feel again, reconnect with purpose, and reclaim their relationships.

"I used to think vulnerability was weakness. Now I know it's my greatest leadership tool."

Marina's Metamorphosis:
From Miscarriage to Movement

Marina's invisible pain was the miscarriage she never told anyone about. It spiraled into depression, self-blame, and disconnection from her partner. Her alchemy began when she joined a grief circle and wrote a letter to the baby she lost. That one act birthed a blog, a book, and now a nonprofit supporting women through silent loss.

"My pain wasn't my prison—it became my platform."

Elena and Marcus:
The Couple Who Chose Conscious Recovery

After infidelity, Elena and Marcus didn't end their marriage—they reinvented it. Through therapy, ayahuasca ceremonies, and brutal honesty, they rebuilt a relationship rooted in truth. Pain became their shared teacher.

"Our marriage ended. But what we built after that was a sacred partnership."

PART IV: THE INVITATION — STEP INTO YOUR UNSTOPPABLE POWER

You've read the chapters. You've seen the patterns. You've likely seen *yourself* in these pages.

Now comes the choice: do you go back to who you were before this journey? Or do you become the version of yourself who was born from the fire?

Living unstoppable isn't about being perfect. It's about being **present**. Being **whole**. Being **awake**.

This is your final invitation.

You are not broken. You are becoming.
You are not behind. You are right on time.
You are not too late. The world is just getting ready for you.

YOUR NEW CREED:

- I honor my scars as symbols of strength.
- I forgive myself for not knowing what I didn't know.
- I live boldly, love deeply, and rest unapologetically.
- I rise—not in spite of my pain, but *because* of it.

INTEGRATION EXERCISES

EXERCISE 1:
NAME THE ASHES, NAME THE GOLD

Prompt:

- What pain or event brought you to your knees?
- What did it teach you?
- What has it made possible?

Take 20 minutes. Write. Feel. No filter.

EXERCISE 2:
RESILIENCE RITUAL MAPPING

Build your daily power rituals:

- Morning: What is one grounding or energizing practice you commit to?
- Midday: What boundary will you uphold today?
- Evening: What will you do to release or reflect?

Write them down and place them where you can see them daily.

EXERCISE 3:
THE UNSTOPPABLE DECLARATION

Write your own declaration. Start with:

"I am no longer waiting for permission to rise. I am…"

Finish the sentence. Add 10 more. Say them aloud in the mirror. Daily.

FINAL WORDS

Whether you are a woman reclaiming her story, or a man rewriting his emotional code—this book was written for *you*. The one who knows there's more. The one who won't settle for survival. The one who is ready to rise.

You are not who you once were. And thank God for that.

Because what rises from the ashes... is unstoppable.

> *"She remembered who she was. And the game changed."*
> — LALAH DELIA

Or as the modern masculine might say:

> *"A man who feels deeply becomes a man who leads authentically."*

The time is now.
The fire is lit.

Welcome to your next chapter.

BONUS CHAPTERS
THE BOARDROOM QUEEN

"I'm a great believer in luck, and I find the harder I work, the more I have of it."
—Thomas Jefferson

BONUS STORY: THE BOARDROOM QUEEN

I wasn't new to pressure.

I had built my entire professional life inside the eye of the storm—leading teams, closing deals, holding space for others while barely holding myself together. But this day was different. It was the kind of day my body warned me about three days in advance—the ache behind my ribs, the nausea that curled around my spine, and the sense of disconnection that came with every shallow breath.

Still, the calendar didn't care. The pitch was scheduled. The execs were flying in. And I had learned long ago that success rarely waited for pain to pass.

I stood in front of the mirror that morning, my reflection catching the bags under my eyes. They weren't from crying. They were from years of pretending everything was fine. I pressed a hot compress to my abdomen while going over my slides. Each movement was calculated, every breath measured.

"Be undeniable," I whispered to myself, applying lipstick like armor.

The conference room was cold, the kind of sterile chill that worked against my pain. My assistant offered me coffee. I declined—my stomach was already doing cartwheels. Instead, I leaned on breathwork. Four counts in, six counts out. "I've done this before," I reminded myself. "I can do it again."

But this wasn't just about getting through the meeting. This was about visibility. Influence. Funding.

And so I did what she always did: delivered. My voice didn't waver once. My eyes scanned the room with poise and control. The deck unfolded seamlessly, and with every passing slide, I could feel the room leaning in.

What they saw: a commanding woman in a navy suit, the epitome of confidence. What they didn't see: the cramp gripping my side like a vice, the sweat pooling at the base of my back, the quiet plea running in my head: "Please let me make it through without fainting."

The Q&A went over time. My smile didn't falter. Neither did my legs—though they begged me to sit.

I shook hands, accepted congratulations, and excused myself with grace. When the boardroom door finally closed behind me, I walked calmly to the restroom, locked the stall, and collapsed onto the closed toilet lid, exhaling a single sentence that had become my ritual:

"I'm proud of you."

Not because I pretended. But because I delivered truth cloaked in elegance. Because my body may have betrayed me, but my spirit never did.

That night, I ordered soup and sat in bed with a heating pad and my journal. My win wasn't just professional. It was spiritual.

Reflections from My Day

Pain doesn't always knock loudly. Sometimes, it whispers through a clenched jaw and unsteady legs. But when we show up anyway—not to fake perfection, but to honor our purpose—we give others permission to redefine power.

That day, I wasn't just a professional. I was a warrior. And if no one clapped when I exited the room, I clapped for myself.

Because power isn't about who sees you—it's about who you are when no one's watching.

Part Two: The Unseen Hours

The night before the pitch, I had barely slept. My body always seemed to know when something big was coming, like it was trying to sabotage my momentum. I had spent hours tossing between heating pads and prayer, half rehearsing, half negotiating with my nervous system.

There was a time in my life when I believed I had to choose—either heal or hustle. Not both. But now I knew: healing *was* the hustle. Showing up *was* the strategy.

Back in my hotel room after the pitch, my inbox was buzzing—thank you notes, a LinkedIn message from a Fortune 100 exec, a request to speak on a women-in-leadership panel. All because I held my power when my body tried to surrender it.

I sat quietly on the edge of the bed, shoes off, feet sore, but spirit steady. I had one hand on my belly and the other on my journal. My handwriting was messy, but my message was clear:

"Today I proved I could be soft and still win. Pain didn't define me. Poise did."

Part Three: Behind the Scenes

What they didn't see was how I prepared for that meeting.
- The playlist I listened to while curling my hair— songs that made me feel like Beyoncé with a mission.
- The raw smoothie I drank instead of breakfast because my stomach was unpredictable.
- The silent gratitude I whispered for even having a voice that mattered in rooms like these.

I remembered what it was like years earlier—when my symptoms first appeared and doctors told me, "It's probably just stress."

I remembered when an old boss called me "too emotional" for leaving early during a flare.

I remembered wondering if I was imagining it all.

But this day—this pitch—was different. Because now I knew the truth.

I wasn't broken. I was *becoming.*

And the version of me that showed up in that boardroom?

I wasn't pretending to be powerful. I *was* powerful. Even in the pain.

Part Four: The Red Bottom Heels

The red bottom heels I wore that day weren't just fashion. They were a promise.

A promise that no matter how much it hurt, I would keep walking.

A promise to myself that power doesn't come from the absence of pain—but from the decision to rise with it.

A promise that I would never again shrink my story to make others comfortable.

I wore them with pride.

Because they weren't just shoes. They were symbols.

Of the woman who leads. The woman who bleeds. And the woman who rises anyway.

My Reflection

There's nothing weak about managing pain in silence.

Leadership isn't always loud. Sometimes it's a whisper in the dark:

"You've got this."

Sometimes it's a quiet cry in a bathroom stall after holding the room for two hours straight.

And sometimes, it's just showing up—when everything in your body says not to.

You don't owe anyone a performance of perfection.

But you owe yourself the truth:

You are more than your pain.

You are a leader. A force. A miracle in motion.

Part Five: The Breakdown Before the Breakthrough

Years earlier, I had a very different kind of meeting. It was my first major leadership presentation—an opportunity that could have fast-tracked my promotion. The night before, my endometriosis symptoms erupted in full force. I called in sick. The deal was reassigned.

My manager at the time—a woman I once admired—shrugged and said, "If you can't handle the heat, maybe leadership isn't your lane."

I went home that day feeling like my body had failed me. Like I had failed myself.

I didn't cry until I saw a little girl on TV giving a speech at a school fundraiser. The girl said, "When I grow up, I want to be a boss who helps people." Something clicked.

*What if your pain isn't the disqualifier?

What if it's the curriculum?

From that day on, I vowed: I wouldn't just rise. I would make space for others to rise too.

Part Six: The Whisper

The morning after the boardroom pitch, I sat at my favorite café. A quiet corner by the window. I wrapped my hands around a warm mug, body aching but soul alive.

An older woman approached my table. "Excuse me," she said. "Were you in the Carter meeting yesterday?" I nodded cautiously.

The woman smiled. "I've worked there 27 years. I've never seen anyone command that room with so much softness and certainty at the same time."

I blinked, taken aback.

"I hope you're the future," the woman said.

I didn't say anything at first. Then: "I'm just trying to build the kind of leadership I never saw."

Final Reflection: The Journal Entry

That night, I wrote:

> *"You don't have to feel perfect to be powerful.*
> *You don't have to be pain-free to be persuasive.*
> *And you don't owe anyone an explanation for how you carry your fire.*
> *All that matters is you keep walking—with truth in your step and purpose in your pulse."*

ENDO-FRIENDLY ANTI-INFLAMMATORY NUTRITION GUIDE

(Gluten-Free • Dairy-Limited • Low Nightshades)

This food approach combines the healing principles of the Mediterranean diet with targeted modifications to reduce inflammation, support digestion, and minimize food sensitivities. It's designed for individuals dealing with chronic pain, autoimmune issues, endometriosis, or hormonal imbalance. I've had my Nutritional Therapist Certification for a decade and through trial and error, this diet works best for me – to avoid endo belly and minimize autoimmune symptoms. If you need help or have questions please feel free to schedule a 1/1 consultation.

🌿 CORE PRINCIPLES

- **Anti-Inflammatory:**
  Focus on whole, nutrient-dense, antioxidant-rich foods.

- **Gluten-Free:**
  Avoid wheat, barley, rye, and processed foods containing gluten.

- **Low Nightshades:**
  Limit or avoid tomatoes, potatoes, peppers, and eggplant (common inflammation triggers for some).

- **Dairy-Limited:**
  Choose non-dairy or low-lactose options; avoid conventional cow's milk products.

- **Mediterranean-Inspired:**
  Emphasize omega-3 fats, lean proteins, fiber-rich veggies, and herbs.

✅ WHAT TO INCLUDE

🥬 VEGETABLES (LOW-NIGHTSHADE FOCUS)

- Leafy greens (kale, spinach, arugula, Swiss chard)
- Cruciferous veggies (broccoli, cauliflower, Brussels sprouts)
- Zucchini, cucumbers, squash
- Carrots, beets, fennel
- Sweet potatoes (in moderation)
- Artichokes, celery, asparagus

🥩 PROTEIN

- Wild-caught fatty fish (salmon, sardines, mackerel)
- Organic, pasture-raised poultry
- Grass-fed beef or lamb (in moderation)
- Eggs (if tolerated)
- Legumes and lentils (watch if you're sensitive to lectins)
- Organic tofu or tempeh (occasionally, for plant-based eaters but do not recommend too much tofu in your diet)

🥥 HEALTHY FATS

- Extra virgin olive oil (primary oil)
- Avocados and avocado oil
- Raw nuts and seeds (chia, flax, pumpkin, walnuts, almonds)
- Omega-3-rich foods (chia, flax, hemp seeds, oily fish)

🍓 FRUITS (LOW GLYCEMIC)

- Berries (blueberries, strawberries, raspberries)
- Stonefruit (apricots, peaches, necatrines)
- Apples, pears, citrus fruits
- Pomegranate, kiwi
- Avoid high-sugar tropical fruits (limit bananas, pineapple, mango)

🌿 GLUTEN-FREE WHOLE GRAINS & STARCHES

- Quinoa, millet, buckwheat, teff
- Wild rice, black rice
- Gluten-free oats
- Root vegetables: parsnips, turnips

🧂 HERBS & SPICES (NATURAL ANTI-INFLAMMATORIES)

- Turmeric + black pepper
- Ginger
- Parsley, oregano, thyme, basil, mint
- Garlic and onion (if tolerated)
- Cinnamon, rosemary

🥥 DAIRY ALTERNATIVES

- Unsweetened almond, coconut, or macadamia milk
- Sheep or goat cheese (in small amounts, if tolerated better than cow's milk)
- Coconut yogurt (unsweetened, with probiotics)

✗ WHAT TO LIMIT OR AVOID

NIGHTSHADES (IF SENSITIVE)

- Tomatoes and tomato-based products
- White and red potatoes
- Eggplant
- Peppers (bell, chili, paprika, cayenne)

INFLAMMATORY FOODS

- Processed/refined oils (canola, soybean, corn)
- Fried foods and fast food
- Refined sugar and artificial sweeteners
- Gluten-containing grains (wheat, barley, rye)
- Processed/packaged snacks

DAIRY

- Conventional milk, cheese, yogurt, butter (organic yogurt and butter can be consumed occasionally & focus on consuming goat and sheep's cheese)
- Ice cream, sour cream, and other full-fat cow dairy

🍵 BEVERAGES

- Filtered water (aim for 2+ liters/day)
- Herbal teas (ginger, peppermint, chamomile, dandelion)
- Green tea or matcha
- Bone broth (great for gut and joint health)
- Limit caffeine and alcohol (especially wine if sensitive to sulfites and honestly, try do go alcohol-free entirely)

"**Disclaimer:** *This guide is for educational purposes only and is not intended to diagnose, treat, cure, or prevent any disease. Everyone's body and lifestyle is unique. Always consult with your healthcare provider or a registered nutritionist before making dietary changes.*"

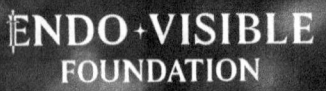

The Endo-Visible Foundation is empowering women with endometriosis to rise, connect, and be heard.

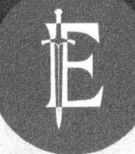

OUR MISSION

To break the silence and stigma surrounding endometriosis by empowering individuals with knowledge, support, and community. Through storytelling, advocacy, and visibility, we strive to uplift those affected and drive meaningful change in how endometriosis is understood and treated.

WHY "ENDO-VISIBLE"?

Endometriosis is often called the invisible disease by the World Health Organization (WHO)—its pain hidden beneath the surface, its impact misunderstood, and those who suffer from it too often unheard.

www.endo-visible.com   endo_visible

We chose the name Endo-Visible Foundation because our mission is to change that. We exist to make endo seen, to give voice to the millions living with this chronic, life-altering condition, and to build a world where women's pain is no longer ignored.

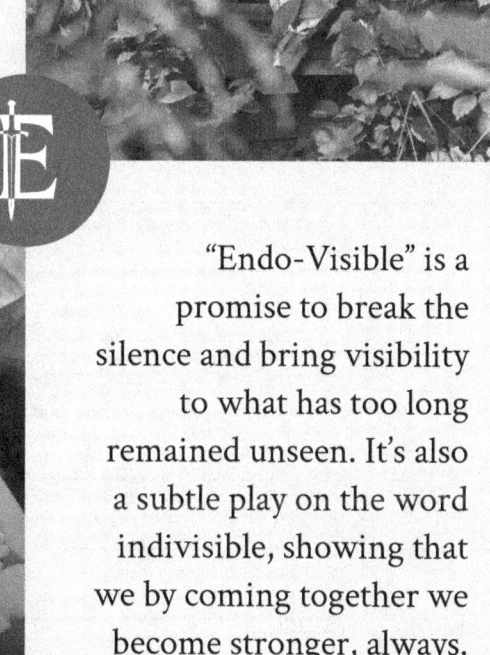

"Endo-Visible" is a promise to break the silence and bring visibility to what has too long remained unseen. It's also a subtle play on the word indivisible, showing that we by coming together we become stronger, always.

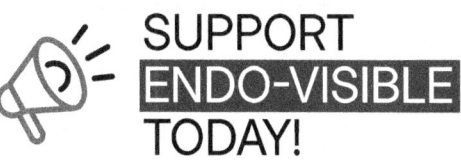  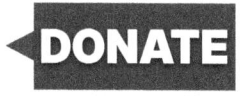

Your donation directly supports education, advocacy, and community-based initiatives that uplift millions of women living with endometriosis.

 donations@endo-visible.com   www.endo-visible.com

GRATITUDE / NOTES

GRATITUDE / NOTES

GRATITUDE / NOTES

GRATITUDE / NOTES

GRATITUDE / NOTES

GRATITUDE / NOTES

GRATITUDE / NOTES

GRATITUDE / NOTES

ABOUT THE AUTHOR

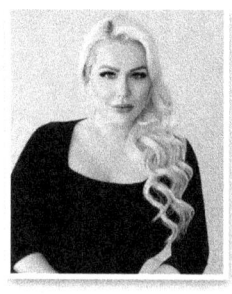 Katya Karlova is a transformational leader, curve model, content creator, and keynote speaker whose journey from corporate executive to creative visionary has inspired thousands worldwide. Formerly an award-winning Vice President of Talent & HR for a billion-dollar health and wellness company, Katya now channels her voice into advocacy, storytelling, and powerful reinvention.

Born in the Republic of Moldova, Katya's early life ignited her passion for human rights and social justice. A proud UCLA graduate (in just three years), she went on to study at NYU, University College London, and was awarded the prestigious Erasmus Mundus Scholarship for her research on human trafficking—an issue close to her heart and homeland.

She is the founder of "EndoVisible" (www.endo-visible.com), a not-for-profit organization dedicated to raising awareness and driving global advocacy for those suffering with endometriosis and other invisible illnesses.

Her accomplishments span boardrooms and stages alike, including:
- 2019 UCLA Young Alumnus of the Year
- 2020 UCLA International Institute Commencement Speaker
- 2022 Top 50 Talent Acquisition Professionals in the U.S.
- 2024 Womenpreneur's Top 20 Most Empowering Women in the U.S.

Now a trailblazing curve model and sought-after voice on healing and empowerment, Katya uses her platform to shed light on invisible illness, emotional resilience, and feminine power.

Her debut book, *Invisible Pain, Unstoppable Power*, is a deeply personal and unapologetically raw exploration of living with undiagnosed endometriosis—and rising beyond it. It is a rallying cry for every woman who has ever been dismissed, gaslit, or underestimated. Through it, Katya invites readers to reclaim their voice, their story, and their unstoppable power.

Katya continues to break barriers, champion self-expression, and speak for those still finding their words. Her mission is clear: to turn invisible pain into undeniable purpose.

Katya Karlova

www.ingramcontent.com/pod-product-compliance
Lightning Source LLC
Chambersburg PA
CBHW060954230426
43665CB00015B/2190